Smashing Idols: Transform Your Body, Mind, and Spirit with a Plant-Based Lifestyle

BY JAYNE M. BOOTH

Unless otherwise noted, all Scripture is taken from the HOLY BIBLE, NEW INTERNATIONAL VERSION, Copyright 1973,1978,1984 by International Bible Society. Used by permission of Zondervan. All rights reserved.

To all who are praying for a solution to your struggle
with weight and its resulting health issues,
May you find the answer to your prayers
within these pages.

First, I would like to thank the Father, Son, and Holy Spirit for guiding me in my search for improved health and directing me to experts who could advise me on my quest. To name a few whose writings, podcasts, and webinars have enlightened me: T. Colin Campbell PhD, Caldwell J. Esselstyn Jr. MD, John McDougall MD, Michael Greger MD, Rev. George H. Malkmus, and John Robbins.

I would also like to personally thank Pastors Bryan Koch, Scott Kramer, Jason James, and Don James who have invited me to share the wholefood plant-based lifestyle with their people. The concern of these ministers for the physical, as well as the spiritual, health of their congregations has been inspiring. A special thank you to Pastor Bryan Koch, who read the very first draft of Smashing Idols, and whose vision encouraged me to publish.

A huge thank you to Christen Bouffard for her exceptional cover design and formatting talents that brought this book to life. You are the best!

I will be eternally grateful to my husband, Dave, my greatest supporter, willing food critic, rock to lean on, shoulder to cry on, and 24/7 in-house IT Department.
Thank you, Dear.

And finally, Christy, Aaron, Alex, Shannon, Ted and Danielle, my faithful cheerleaders in all things food related.
I love you all!

DISCLAIMER

The health information in this book is based on the Bible, the author's personal experience, and research. The author is neither diagnosing nor prescribing treatment. It is recommended that the reader inform their doctor about any changes to diet or lifestyle they intend to pursue.

If you are taking prescription medications, it is doubly important that a healthcare professional monitor your progress, because positive
physical changes can occur rather rapidly as you lose weight. Only you are responsible for your diet and healthcare decisions, so note any changes in symptoms and discuss them with your provider.

Your doctor may need to adjust or eliminate medications as your general health improves.

Copyright ©2021 by Jayne M. Booth

Smashing Idols: Transform Your Body, Mind, and Spirit with a Plant-Based Lifestyle

All rights reserved. No part of this publication may be reproduced, distributed, or transmitted in any form or by any means, including photocopying, recording, or other electronic or mechanical methods, without prior written permission of the publisher, except in the case of brief quotations embodied in critical reviews and certain other noncommercial uses permitted by copyright law.

Although the author and publisher have made every effort to ensure that the information in this book was correct at press time, the author and publisher do not assume and herby disclaim any liability to any party for any loss, damage, or disruption caused by errors or omissions, whether such errors or omissions result from negligence, accident, or any other cause.

Adherence to all applicable laws and regulations, including international, federal, state, and local governing professional licensing, business practices, advertising, and all other aspects of doing business in the US, Canada or any other jurisdiction is the sole responsibility of the reader and consumer.

Neither the author nor the publisher assumes any responsibility or liability whatsoever on behalf of the consumer or reader of this material. Any perceived slight of any individual or organization is purely unintentional.

The resources in this book are provided for informational purposes only and should not be used to replace the specialized training and professional judgement of a health care or mental health care professional.

Neither the author nor the publisher can be held responsible for the use of the information provided within this book. Please always consult a trained professional before making any decision regarding treatment of yourself or others.

Copyright ©2021 by Jayne M. Booth

Smashing Idols: Transform Your Body, Mind, and Spirit with a Plant-Based Lifestyle

ISBN: 978-1-7375864-1-8

LCCN: 2021917623

Contents

DAY 1 – MY STORY 13
I John 5:21
    BATTLE PLAN 17

DAY 2 – CENTER YOUR LIFE 19
Psalm 118:8
    JUICING 22

DAY 3 – YOUR TENDENCY IS NOT YOUR DESTINY 23
2 Timothy 1:7
    GRAZE 27

DAY 4 – WHICH PATH 29
Matthew 7:13, 14
    MOVE 33

DAY 5 – HIS PRECIOUS CHILD 35
1 Corinthians 6:19, 20
    HEALTHY SNACKS EVEN A CHILD CAN PREPARE 38

DAY 6 – TRUTH OR CONSEQUENSES 39
Proverbs 1:20-22
    SEVEN ACTION STEPS TOWARD WISE EATING 42

DAY 7 – FATHER KNOWS BEST 43
Job 28:20-28
    DAD'S TEX-MEX BEANS 47

DAY 8 – THE KING IS WATCHING 49
Daniel 1:8, 11-18, 20
    DANIEL'S WINNING STRATEGY 53

DAY 9 – YOUR TALENT 55
Matthew 25:14-30
    SAMPLE FOOD JOURNAL PAGE* 61

Contents (cont.)

DAY 10 – SNAKES AMONG US **63**
Numbers 21:4-9
    CABBAGE WALDORF SALAD (FOR A CROWD) 66

DAY 11 – THE SECRET **67**
Psalm 92:12-15
    PRAYER OF SUBMISSION AND RELIANCE ON GOD 70

DAY 12 – THE STOMACH GOD **71**
Philippians 3:18-19
    SIMPLE "GREEN GOODNESS" SALAD DRESSING 74

DAY 13 – FOOD TO DIE FOR **75**
Proverbs: 9:11, 17-18
    INNOCENT ICE CREAM 78

DAY 14 – KEEP YOUR EYES ON THE PRIZE **79**
Jeremiah 32:31, 33-34
    NO-BAKE GRANOLA BARS 82

DAY 15 – DON'T DIET IN A DONUT SHOP **83**
James 1:14-15
    COCONUTTY "DONUT HOLES" 85

DAY 16 – PLAN YOUR WAY OUT **87**
1 Corinthians 10:13
    BASIC HUMMUS 91

DAY 17 – BLESS THE BEASTS **93**
Exodus 23:5, 11-12
    GRILLED NO-BEEF BURGER 97

DAY 18 – YOUR WELL **99**
Proverbs 4:23
    HEART-HEALTHY RICE AND BEANS 102

Contents (cont.)

DAY 19 - THE CHOICE IS YOURS 103
Psalm 78:18, 29-31
    TIPS FOR HEALTHY EATING WHEN DINING OUT 106

DAY 20 - CONFESSION OF TRANSGRESSION............ 109
Psalm 32:1-5
    PRAYER OF CONFESSION*......................... 112

DAY 21 - YOUR BODY, GOD'S TEMPLE 113
1 Corinthians 3:16-17
    CLEAN OUT YOUR PANTRY AND REFRIGERATOR......... 116

DAY 22 - THE PROVERBS 31 WIFE...................... 119
Proverbs 31:14-15, 26-27
    EGG SUBSTITUTIONS 122

DAY 23 - COUNT YOUR BLESSINGS..................... 123
Psalm 4:8
    FOR MORE INFORMATION ABOUT SLEEP 126

DAY 24 - LORDSHIP 127
Romans 14:2-4, 17-18
    NINJA TUNA SALAD 131

DAY 25 - YOUR DAILY BREAD 133
Ezekiel 4:9
    OVERNIGHT CHAI STEEL-CUT OATS.................. 136

DAY 26 - THE BEST MEDICINE 137
Proverbs 17:22
    LAUGH YOUR WAY TO HEALTH...................... 140

DAY 27 - CONFORM OR TRANSFORM................... 141
Romans 12:1-2
    TAKE THE INITIATIVE 144

Contents (cont.)

DAY 28 - HONEY DOS AND DONT'S **145**
Proverbs 24:13, 25:16,27
    HONEY AS MEDICINE. 148
DAY 29 - SHOPPING IN THE GARDEN. **149**
Proverbs 6:6-8, 30:25
    HOW TO FREEZE RAW TOMATOES. 152
DAY 30 - BLOSSOM! BLOOM! GROW!. **153**
Galatians 5:16, 22-24
    SELF-CONTROL AT THE DINNER TABLE. 156
DAY 31 - HIS BENEFITS FOR OUR BENEFIT **157**
Psalm 103:2-5
    APPLE PIE SMOOTHIE. 160
    SAMPLE FOOD JOURNAL PAGE. 161
    SAMPLE FOOD JOURNAL PAGE. 162
    SAMPLE FOOD JOURNAL PAGE. 163
    SAMPLE FOOD JOURNAL PAGE. 164
    SAMPLE FOOD JOURNAL PAGE. 165
    SAMPLE FOOD JOURNAL PAGE. 166
    SAMPLE FOOD JOURNAL PAGE. 167

For more recipes, restaurant reviews, and tips for living a healthy plant-based lifestyle, follow the author at vegtutor.com.

Day 1 - My Story

I John 5:21
Dear children keep yourselves from idols.

A woman my age. A woman MY age? I was only in my forties, not my eighties. Was it all going to be downhill from here...ALREADY?

I drove away from the doctor's office going over everything he had said. "Your body has served you well all these years, but you can expect to feel some aches and pains now. It's all part of the aging process. This is normal for a woman your age."

I knew I was carrying some extra weight from baby number four, who was already in elementary school. My yearly bouts of the flu and winter colds proved that my immune system was not what it should be. But it was the exhausting lack of energy that had forced me to make an appointment with our family doctor.

In over two decades of marriage and four children, I had never had trouble managing the hectic schedules of our family. I was a professional volunteer: classroom mother, field trip chaperone, bake sale contributor, craft sale chairperson, Sunday school and VBS teacher—name a committee and I've probably served on it. When the school bus pulled up in the afternoon, I put on my "Expert Carpool Driver hat" and ferried our children and their friends to and from music and dance lessons, play practices, sports practices, games and meets, Girl Scouts, Boy Scouts, part-time jobs, parties, and sleepovers.

It was a crazy busy life, but I loved it...until now. Now my body was screaming for attention. (Maybe you know how that feels). I remembered what healthy felt like, and this was not it. I thought my doctor would have some reasonable answers for my lack of energy and shortness of breath when climbing the stairs. I wanted him to have a better explanation than just growing old. I wanted a solution. There had to be one. Instead, he slid a prescription for Valium across his desk and said, "It's time to slow down." Stunned, I looked at the prescription and slowly slid it back toward the doctor. No! I decided I would have to find the answers to my health problems on my own. So began my quest. I started studying everything the experts had to say about health and healing. I read the latest medical research articles and dozens of books and spent hours on the Internet searching for clues and taking notes. I prayed every day that God would direct me to the information I needed. Instinctively knowing that the answer to every question in life is buried somewhere in the wisdom of God's Word, I dug into the scriptures harder than ever before, searching.

As I prayed, and as I read, one common theme seemed to emerge from all my study: a natural, whole-food, plant-based diet and lifestyle. This was a surprise to me. I had always associated vegetarians with New-Age spirituality, cults, and Peace Corps volunteers. Could God be telling me, a middle-aged Christian woman, to become a vegetarian? Really, God? I did not want to believe that I had allowed my appetite, my stomach, to become a god. It took two years of collecting evidence before I finally surrendered and agreed that this was indeed the Lord's leading and will. I did not love vegetables. A plant-based lifestyle was not a change this lifelong carnivore was eager to embrace, but I knew it was time to smash that idol.

In addition, I had a husband and family to convince. Since I did all the cooking in our house, if I became a vegetarian, everybody would become vegetarians...at least when they ate at home. My husband assured me that if the food was delicious, he would eat it. I'm sure

Dave thought this was all just a passing phase, and if he went along with it, in a couple of weeks life would return to normal. With his blessing, I immediately signed up for a vegetarian cooking class. In that six weeks, I discovered a whole new world of food I had never experienced! Cooking became an adventure instead of a routine chore. With only a few complaints, my family obligingly sampled and critiqued each meal as I experimented with new recipes and exotic ingredients. Some recipes were keepers, and the dog happily gobbled up the rejects. Our daughter's friend once remarked, "I love to eat at your house because I never know what to expect!" They really were good sports during my learning process.

As I changed the way I was eating from the Standard American Diet (SAD) to the healthy diet God was showing me, my tastes began to change also. After a few months, my desire for meat was completely gone. Heavily processed junk food was no longer appealing because I began to enjoy the flavor of God's whole, natural plant foods more. (For example, today when I pass a fast-food restaurant the aroma of beef on the grill is not appetizing at all. It smells like greasy dirt to me!) When I stopped gorging on junk food I expected to lose some weight, but I was surprised how quickly and easily my body started to shed excess pounds and replace them with the energy I had been missing for so long.

There is no way to describe feeling clean on the inside, but that is exactly how I felt as my body slimmed down and was cleansed from years of toxic overload due to a diet of processed fake foods and fatty animal products. I started to believe that maybe I could do this. I was so excited when my weight began to drop three pounds per week that I promised myself new clothes if I lost fifteen pounds. Well, I got to do that TWICE in only three months of eating a whole food, mostly vegan diet! That is no meat, no eggs, no dairy, and no junk food. It is the original diet God gave to Adam and Eve in the Garden of Eden. After three months, the weight loss slowed until I finally stabilized at my normal weight, thirty-five energy-draining pounds less than when I started just five months earlier. This whole process was a science experiment (because I still was testing God to see if this truly was from Him), and I was the "lab rat," but as the evidence mounted, I had to conclude that feeling good is just more satisfying than eating the SAD. Eating the old way was never best, and my body had been telling me that. What amazed me was that it didn't require any special diet program, pills, or expensive prepackaged meals. God's diet doesn't cost anything except for the healthy food, and you have to buy food anyway. Even my husband lost ten pounds and lowered his cholesterol and blood pressure by just living with me—imagine that! He was sold.

As we both lost weight, our walks became hikes. We bought bicycles and started to enjoy new hobbies together like canoeing and ballroom dance classes. Without all that extra weight to carry around, I not only had more energy and fewer aches and pains, I actually felt younger!

It has been twenty years since the Lord directed me away from the world's diet to a whole-food plant-based diet. In that time, God continued to lead and teach me. I discovered that the Bible is filled with words of health and healing, hidden in plain sight, where I never noticed them before. I began to teach others.

Have you been praying about your health or your weight? Maybe God is answering that prayer right now, so don't wait. Embrace the adventure! You will have to smash some idols along the way. Are you up to the challenge? This will be a period of physical and spiritual growth, but you will emerge victorious with a stronger body, a stronger character, and a stronger testimony. God bless you on your journey!

BATTLE PLAN

This book is designed to be a daily call to action—an encouragement for all believers as we walk the path to maturity, striving to honor God in every area, including our bodies. I hope you will join me on this physical and spiritual adventure to better health. The benefits are priceless. Please take a few minutes at the beginning of each day to read one chapter of Smashing Idols. My prayer is that what you read in the morning will give you confidence that a healthy physical body is God's will, and that confidence will encourage you to take some free and natural steps to make it happen for you. I thank God every day that He answers prayer. He not only saved my soul, but He also saved my body from years of being sick, tired, and overweight. Thank you, Lord!

Day 2 - Center Your Life

Psalm 118:8
It is better to take refuge in the Lord than to trust in man.

    The Bible is a collection of sixty-six separate and complete books, all authored by God but written by forty different men, each inspired by the Holy Spirit to record the very mind and heart of our Creator. It is awesome to consider the wisdom contained in scripture: guidance, encouragement, and life lessons designed to address every topic under the sun. Every word in the 31,103 verses in the Bible originated with God and has a divine purpose in the life of a believer. It is no accident that God placed Psalm 118:8 in the very center of His Holy Word. This central Bible verse is God ordained to be the key anchor verse upon which to center your life. As a person seeking to live a life that honors and pleases God, you must examine and compare all your thoughts, actions, and motives against the Lord's wisdom. This is why it is so important to spend some prime time every day reading and meditating on God's Word. I would recommend starting each morning by investigating what God has to say first before the cacophony of daily modern life bombards your mind with the distracting media buzz that drones on and on until your final yawn of the evening.

    On the subject of health, it's impossible to avoid the negative input that assaults our senses from every source. Newspaper, radio, billboards, Internet, magazines, television, statisticians, health professionals, and "experts" all seem to spew dire health reports concerning product and drug recalls, this or that weight loss plan, vitamin deficiencies, new and exotic diseases, epidemics, birth defects, the physical degeneration of aging, prescribed medical tests and routine lab work you must have done or else...but nothing ever changes. It's so confusing! Do you live in quiet desperation because the more you learn the more helpless you feel? Do you really have no control over your own body? Are you just another victim in a game of chance, waiting for the dreaded diagnosis to strike if your number is called?

My doctor told me that my symptoms were "normal for a woman your age." This seems to be the prevailing thought in modern healthcare: sooner or later you will be in pain; you will be sick; it's just a matter of time—but don't worry, we have a pill for that. Do you want to trust your health to this world's conflicted, confusing system? Do you want to survive on handfuls of prescribed or OTC medications that merely mask the symptoms, but never address the cause?

I have good news for you! God's Word has plenty to say about the care and health of the human body. It's all simple, free, and you can do it yourself, but first, you have to decide whether you will "take refuge in the Lord" or "trust in man." Psalm 118:8, the central verse of the Bible, tells us it is better to trust God and His Word in every area of life—this includes health. Should you throw away all your prescription medications and just pray about your health? No! That would be foolish. (Never make a medication change without your physician's approval.) It is my hope and prayer that as you read and meditate on one chapter of this book each day, God will open your heart and mind to the many free and natural ways He prescribes to affect and protect your physical health. After all, God designed your body, so who would know better how to care for it?

As you learn and put into practice God's natural principles for a healthy body, mind, and spirit, you will gain a new appreciation for the miraculous healing potential the Creator has programmed into man's cell. Don't be surprised when your body starts to respond to all the good changes you're making to help it get strong and healthy. It won't happen all at once. Remember, it took years for you to get worn down and plumped up, so it will take some time to undo the damage, but be faithful. Your doctor may soon be telling YOU that he is going to reduce or eliminate some of your medications—that's exciting!

If you center your life on Psalm 118:8 and trust God's natural wisdom for health, you will be doing everything you can to cooperate with your body's own healing processes by promoting an environment for enduring health. You will notice the changes as they start to occur. Others will begin to comment, "You look different—have you lost weight?" "You look great!" "Why, you're absolutely glowing!" Just tell them that you made one quality decision, to center your life, and that changed everything. They will ask what that means—what a testimony!

BATTLE PLAN
JUICING

Try juicing at home. Pure carrot/apple juice is a refreshing nutrient boost on your journey to health and healing. Green juices and carrot juice are concentrated nutrition aimed straight at your hungry cells. Add half an apple for a little zing! Try to make fresh juice (not bottled) part of your daily routine.

If you juice first thing every morning, then you won't forget to do it. Make enough for two servings so one juice is ready and waiting for you in the afternoon or when you get home from work. Then you'll be able to concentrate on preparing a healthy dinner instead of your growling stomach.

Don't feel that you have to rush right out and buy a big expensive juicer before you can start this new juicing habit. Use the one you have until it dies or until you can afford a new one. If you don't already have a juicer, then research the different types. You can check the classified ads, Craigslist, and garage sales if cost is an issue. It doesn't have to be expensive as long as it works.

Ease of cleaning is also something to consider. Some are dishwasher safe; some must be washed by hand. The best juicer is the one you will use consistently, so the primary factor is YOU. Start today!

Day 3 - Your Tendency Is Not Your Destiny

2 Timothy 1:7
For God did not give us a spirit of timidity, but a spirit of power, of love and of self-discipline. (NIV)
– For God hath not given us a spirit of fear; but of power, and of love, and of a sound mind. (KJV)

We live in a world of chemically laced, genetically altered, sugar-coated, flavor-enhanced "food" choices. Food recalls because of contamination or safety issues are daily occurrences. An array of modern drugs is available to treat our illnesses, but we often hear of drug recalls, or we simply read the list of drug side effects and wonder if our sickness isn't safer than taking the prescribed medication. In addition, we are bombarded with advice about which medical tests we need. Mammograms, prostate exams, colonoscopies, and PAP tests are just a few of the regular screenings for which Americans anxiously await results. We want to trust our doctors to treat us when we are ill, but they are required to disclose all possible complications and survival rates. After hearing that, we'd really rather just stay out of the doctor's office and away from the hospital if at all possible.

With all this information, and considering each one of these choices, it is easy to become overwhelmed by fear and anxiety about our health. Some people have thrown up their hands in despair. Deciding to ignore everything they see and hear, they say, "My father lived to be ninety eating whatever he wanted, and he never went to the doctor. If that was good enough for him, then it's good enough for me, too!" Others live in dread of their impending physical doom. Knowing their family history, they obsess over their symptoms imagining every ache or pain to be arthritis (like Grandma had) and every pimple a tumor (just like Uncle George's). This resignation to a future of poor health can easily lead to depression which causes its own list of health problems. Please hear this: scientific research is now showing that you can actually turn off hereditary tendencies toward certain diseases by diet and lifestyle changes. You do not need to live in fear!

At this point of confusion in our complicated, information-saturated, modern world, let me remind you that God's ways are simple, and His Word is true. God placed the first man and woman in a garden because in that environment they could easily find everything they needed not only to survive but to thrive (Genesis 1:29). As you walk through your grocery store, try to choose foods you would find living in a garden. Fresh garden produce is THE FOOD your Creator designed specifically for humans to eat—isn't that simple?

It is commonly known that the chlorophyll molecule in plants and the hemoglobin molecule in human blood are very similar—this should be a clue as we decide what to eat. Healthy blood is a sign of a healthy body (that is why doctors rely on blood tests to diagnose illness). Fresh fruits and vegetables are excellent food choices and not only for their vitamin and mineral content; they also contain a synergistic blend of phytonutrients that science still doesn't completely understand, but God does. He designed the foods in the garden to keep us healthy! Man-made vitamin and mineral supplements cannot duplicate the complex nutritional blend in whole foods. Fresh fruits and vegetables are high in pure water, a primary need of every cell in your body. Eaten raw, they contain enzymes that help to digest and distribute nutrients throughout the body. Garden produce is highly alkaline, which greatly reduces the acidity level within the body; inversely, the more cooked foods and the more animal foods you consume the higher the acidity level you will maintain. Acidity causes inflammation which leads to disease. Remember, cancer cannot survive within a healthy, balanced system. What you eat does make a difference.

Organic produce is always best if you have a choice. In the Garden of Eden, there were no chemical fertilizers, herbicides, or pesticides. There were no genetically modified (GMO) crops. We were not created to consume these molecularly modified foods, and they place unnecessary stress on our physical bodies as they try to process them. Originally, all food was organic just the way God designed it: perfect for the nourishment of human beings who lived long and healthy lives as long as they followed God's dietary instructions.

As you strive to choose healthy foods, you can pretty much stay out of the center aisles of the grocery store. The snack foods, processed cereals, dead canned foods, white pasta, and bakery items there provide little, if any, real nutrition. Most are empty calories and actually place a burden on the body as it must work harder to filter through the artificial coloring, acidic sweeteners and fillers, hydrogenated fats, and chemical vitamins (that is what the term "enriched" means) all of which have been added to make these manmade "foods" more appealing to the eye and taste buds.

Love yourself enough to make healthy food choices a priority in your life. Trust God enough to follow His dietary plan. Don't eat to create health problems that promote thoughts of fear and dread of your next doctor visit or lab test results. Choosing a whole-food plant-based diet composed of vegetables, fruits, whole grains, legumes, nuts, and seeds, with the majority raw, is the first step you can take on your path to better health and healing.

God has not given us a spirit of fear. Most of our health worries we create ourselves. He has given us a sound mind, able to discern the good from the bad. You can make excellent food choices. You don't need to accept your family health history as your own fate IF you decide to change generational eating patterns that created that health history in the first place. It's not only diseases that run in families, it's also recipes and eating patterns that are passed from generation to generation. Nothing will change if you don't change something. Your family medical history is only your tendency, not your destiny. Don't live in fear. In faith, you can choose to change, improve your diet, relax, and enjoy better health while following God's original diet.

BATTLE PLAN
GRAZE

If you are just starting to eat healthy, then try for just one meal each day to eat only what you would find in a garden. What would that look like? A crisp colorful salad, a thick cold smoothie (banana, pineapple, and cucumber blended with some ice is a delicious combo), or a plate of juicy cut fruit and a handful of raw almonds or walnuts? These straight-from-the-garden meals require only basic ingredients, and you don't need any cooking experience to prepare a magnificent raw lunch. Be creative. Make it colorful and make it huge!

In addition, you can also make your between-meal snacks nutrient-rich, raw vegetable and fruit treats. This simple routine is a strong foundation for a robust whole-food, plant-based lifestyle that will support health and healing in your entire body.

Day 4- Which Path

Matthew 7:13, 14
Enter through the narrow gate. For wide is the gate and broad is the road that leads to destruction, and many enter through it. But small is the gate and narrow the road that leads to life, and only a few find it.

"Oh, I could never eat like that because: I have to attend too many dinner parties; my husband would never eat that way, and I have to cook for him, too, you know; I have to entertain too many business clients; my wife just doesn't cook that way; my kids would complain; I don't have time to cook healthy meals; exercise just doesn't fit into my schedule; etc., etc., etc... ."What people really mean when they verbalize these excuses is that they are simply not willing to make any changes or to do anything different from their normal routine. It is so much easier to keep doing what you've always done even if it doesn't produce the results you desire...or is it? Your health will not change unless YOU do something different.

If you insist on staying on "the broad road," eating like the rest of the world, then you must also accept the fact that you will reach your chosen destination, which is fatigue, obesity, and sickness in your physical body...just like everyone else who is eating the Standard American Diet. We don't need any more government-sponsored studies or medical research to tell us that we are killing ourselves with our affluent, fast-paced, overindulgent habits.

The evidence of our unhealthy choices in the areas of food and lifestyle is everywhere. Adult-onset diabetes is epidemic and is currently being seen even in children. Can you believe that most American children already have signs of atherosclerosis in their veins and show a need for preventive cardiology in early life?*

As food servings have been super-sized, clothing manufacturers have redesigned (enlarged) their patterns and adjusted the sizing to accommodate, and flatter, the expanding girth of the typical modern consumer. So please don't depend on your pants size to accurately tell if you've gained weight. The old size 12 is the new size 8. You may have gained more inches than you suspect! Drug companies perpetually offer to doctors an ever-growing list of medications to prescribe for their patients who are suffering from the symptoms of modern lifestyle diseases. Drugs only dull the symptoms but do not treat the cause. (And please remember, each prescription comes with its own list of side effects that may also require treatment.) Clearly, we are doing this to ourselves. You cannot eat the world's diet and not expect to suffer the world's illnesses.

Matthew 7:14 talks about a narrow road that leads not to destruction, but to life. We, the church, must snap out of our complacency concerning diet and lifestyle. We cannot blindly continue to follow the world down the widest path available if we want to be effective in the work God has called us to do. If the road you are on is not taking you where you want to go health-wise, then it's time to resolve to get back on the narrow road that leads to life—healthy, vibrant, productive life!

How do you do this? Well, once you have decided to pursue a healthy life, you will want to alter your diet. You will want to eat more raw, whole foods, lots of green leafy vegetables, colorful fresh fruits, whole grains, legumes, nuts, and seeds. When you remove the junk "food" from your diet you will embark on a new adventure in eating and cooking with new recipes (look for them!) that incorporate these nutrient-rich foods into your daily lifestyle. You will stop including animal foods in your diet. All animal foods have way too much fat and no fiber, making them very difficult for your body to process. They place stress on your entire digestive system, causing constipation and weight gain, and initiating illness.

You will also want to include daily exercise, preferably in the fresh air, but in a gym is okay, too, especially if the weather is bad or you need the motivation of working out with a group to keep it interesting. Look for ways to incorporate exercise into your normal routine. Take the stairs instead of the elevator. Park a couple of blocks away from your destination and walk the rest of the way. Join a hiking, biking, or walking club, and enjoy this beautiful world we live in. Instead of lounging on the sofa while watching TV, do some push-ups and sit-ups during this free time. Come on, you're not too tired to exercise; you're too tired because you DON'T exercise!

Lift hand weights. Start small and gradually work up to heavier weights as you get stronger. Keep your weights by your favorite chair in front of the TV, and use them!

Try balancing on one foot to strengthen core muscles and improve your balance and coordination. When you get good at balancing on one foot, try doing it with your eyes closed—that's a challenge! Research shows that lack of balance and coordination are the causes of most adult falls. All of these little physical activities will not only help you to burn calories so that you look and feel better, but they will also strengthen your muscles and bones, helping you to avoid fractures as you age.

On the narrow road to health, purified or bottled spring water—not coffee, tea, soda, or even tap water—will be your main beverage. It is important to drink plenty of pure clean water, particularly now that you are exercising regularly. How much water should you drink? This is a handy formula: take your weight, divide that number in half, and that is how many ounces of water you need daily. (Example: 150 lbs. divided by 2 = 75 oz. of water/day.)

Walking down the narrow road with an arsenal of superfood ideas in place, a more active lifestyle, and plenty of pure water, you will begin to sense renewed energy and strength. You will have a brand-new feeling, too—an awareness of being clean from the inside out. (This feeling is hard to describe, but you will know when it happens.)

Soon you will be sprinting, not merely walking, down the narrow path that leads to life, and you will be encouraging others to join you on the road to better health.

*The 1992 Bogalusa Heart Study, *Eat to Live: the Revolutionary Formula for Fast and Sustained Weight Loss*, by Joel Fuhrman, M.D., Little, Brown, 2005, p. 19

BATTLE PLAN
MOVE

That's it: MOVE! Stand, walk, run! Try reducing the time you spend sitting. No one else can do this for you. Make it a conscious effort, a quest, to find more and more ways to be active in your everyday life. Put your sneakers on first thing in the morning so you're prepared.

Find extra reasons to go up and down the stairs at home. When you're on the phone, walk around the room instead of sitting. Walk instead of driving to nearby destinations. Walk with a friend or neighbor and enjoy chatting while you walk. Move! Do a daily prayer walk through the neighborhood as part of your devotional time with God. Mow your own lawn instead of hiring a service. Sweep the porch, sweep the front steps, sweep the sidewalk, sweep the driveway—just move!

Join a Mall Walkers Club or sign up for an exercise class. You can easily cover a mile or more in climate-controlled comfort (bad weather is no excuse) speed walking through the mall before the shoppers arrive. Don't forget your water!

The more you move the more calories you will burn. You will build strong muscles and bones, reducing the chances that you will suffer bone-breaking falls from osteoporosis in the future. As you become more active and fit, your heart will also grow stronger, and the weight you lose through physical activity will improve the health of every part of your body. So, move. It's up to you to do something different... just MOVE!

Day 5 - His Precious Child

1 Corinthians 6:19, 20

Do you not know that your body is a temple of the Holy Spirit who is in you, whom you received from God? You are not your own; you were bought at a price. Therefore honor God with your body.

I remember one Sunday morning when, as a young mother, I was pulled out of church by an anxious nursery worker who explained that our fourteen-month-old daughter, our firstborn, had fallen and cut her lip. We slipped out the back door of the sanctuary and hurried down the hallway. I could hear Christy's cries growing louder as we neared. Entering the roomful of toddlers, I saw a nursery volunteer holding an ice-filled "boo-boo bunny" against my daughter's swollen split lip as blood and tears dripped down Christy's chin and onto her white pinafore. In an instant, my knees turned to jelly, and I gasped—it was the first time I had ever seen my child bleed, and I will never forget that moment!

Fortunately, my motherly instinct overruled my inclination to faint, and I was able to gather my child into my arms and comfort her until the bleeding stopped and she calmed down. This accident didn't leave even a tiny scar on Christy's face, but the incident is forever etched in my memory.

In that moment, I realized just how precious my child was to me. In that moment, I knew as never before that I didn't want anything to hurt her—ever. I knew that I would always do whatever I could to keep my daughter safe from harm. Then I understood the stories I'd heard about mothers who sacrificed their own lives to save the life of their child. It all made sense to me, and then I understood that I, too, would do anything to protect my child even at the expense of my own life.

And, it was also at that moment that I understood God's love for me. I understood how He could bleed and die for us, His precious children. He loved us so much that He paid the ultimate sacrifice—He gave His very life—so we wouldn't have to suffer. Then our Heavenly Father sealed us into His family by placing His Holy Spirit in our earthly bodies. We are His children, and He will love us forever. Do we appreciate that fact? Do we really understand what it cost Him to save His children, to dwell in us?

If we honestly do understand that we were bought at a price, and we understand the high value of that price, then why do we dishonor God by abusing our physical bodies where His Holy Spirit dwells? If we do comprehend His sacrifice, then we cannot say, "This is my body, and I'll do whatever I want, and I'll eat whatever I want," or "If I don't feel like exercising, then I don't have to." To live our lives according to our own selfish desires is to devalue the death of Christ on the cross. We are commanded to "honor God with our bodies." This isn't optional, it's a command. As harsh as it may sound, to do anything less is disobedience.

Most Christians make the effort to attend church services, sing worship songs, and even strive to maintain some type of daily prayer and Bible reading. These are all good God-honoring habits. However, how are you honoring God in your body? You may say, "Well, I don't smoke or abuse alcohol or drugs." That is commendable, but how are you eating? Everyone eats several times a day, so it is an area where we are all tempted. Is yours a healthy diet? Are you consuming plenty of fresh vegetables and fruit or plenty of super-sized, fatty fast food? Are you drinking pure water and fresh vegetable juices, or energy drinks and colas? A good rule of thumb is: if it can't be grown in a garden then it shouldn't be on your plate.

What are you doing to keep your body physically fit? To maintain health, strength, and balance the human body needs 30-60 minutes of strenuous exercise at least 5 times per week. (Hint: if you're not sweating, then you're not exercising.) If you are lounging on the couch or sitting at the computer for hours at a time, then you are robbing your body of the physical activity it needs to stay strong and healthy. Only physical exercise will build muscle tissue. Your heart is the most important muscle in your body, and you need to keep that most vital muscle strong. Your lymphatic system also requires exercise to function properly so it can remove toxins and enhance your immune system.

To deny your body proper nutrition and adequate exercise is to invite illness into God's temple. Don't try to fool God by asking Him to heal you if you are not willing to do everything you can do, daily, to maintain a strong healthy body. You are His precious child. He loves you more than anything and paid a high price for you. Make the health of your physical body a priority, and you will be rewarded with the strength and vitality you need to serve others and to say, "Thank You" to God for His great love. "You were bought at a price. Therefore, honor God with your body."

BATTLE PLAN
HEALTHY SNACKS EVEN A CHILD CAN PREPARE

- A handful of raw almonds, sunflower seeds, or pumpkin seeds and organic raisins
- Organic apple slices with a couple of tablespoons of almond butter or sunflower seed butter for a dip
- Organic carrot sticks or other raw vegetable sticks or slices with hummus dip
- An apple, pear, banana, or a handful of berries… any whole fruit you like

Take these along with you when you walk the mall, take them to work or school (most will fit in your pocket) so you aren't tempted to stop for ice cream or a soft pretzel.

Day 6 - Truth or Consequenses

Proverbs 1:20-22

Wisdom calls aloud in the street, she raises her voice in the public squares; at the head of the noisy streets she cries out, in the gateways of the city she makes her speech: "How long will you simple ones love your simple ways? How long will mockers delight in mockery and fools hate knowledge?"
Proverbs 1:32 – For the waywardness of the simple will kill them and the complacency of fools destroy them...

News about the benefits of a healthy lifestyle is everywhere: newspapers, magazines, TV, radio, Internet. We are bombarded daily with diet and lifestyle recommendations: eat blueberries for memory acuity, spinach for eye health, flaxseed for Omega 3 fatty acids. We need more Vitamin D, so we are advised to spend 15 minutes each day in the sunshine or take a supplement. A diet high in vegetables and fruits protects us from cancer, heart disease, diabetes, stroke, and on, and on, and on...

The American Cancer Society, the American Heart Association, the American Academy of Pediatrics, the American Dietetic Association, the National Institutes of Health, and the American Society of Clinical Nutrition are all publishing guidelines promoting a diet composed of "mostly fruits and vegetables with very little simple sugar or high-fat foods, especially animal foods." *

With all this information pummeling us every day it is amazing how Americans can tune it all out, yet diligently search the Sunday newspaper for a coupon to a favorite fast-food restaurant. Weekly, we wheel our empty grocery carts straight through the produce aisle on our way to fill it in the meat, bakery, and dairy departments. When we finally push that overloaded cart through the checkout line we don't even realize that much of the contents of the boxes, cans, and cartons on which we have chosen to spend our hard-earned dollars cannot even be called "food" because it will provide little, if any, real nutrition to sustain our bodies and maintain health. Wise shoppers realize that just because it's edible doesn't mean it should be consumed, and just because it's sold in the grocery store doesn't mean it's nutritious. As wise consumers, let's spend more time searching for healthy purchases instead of coupons!

From now on, please try to consider the source and consciously observe the commercial messages around you concerning diet and lifestyle. As you shop wisely, don't depend on slick colorful boxes, labels, and advertisements to help you decide which foods to purchase. Of course, the National Dairy Council is going to tell you to drink more milk—what else would they say? No matter how healthy an industry tells you their product is, remember it's just an ad to make a sale. Industry can find an isolated study to justify just about any claim they want to promote.

When I finally decided to wake up and pay attention, I was astounded by how much dietary recommendations have changed in recent years. Due to the escalation of disease rates in America, advanced scientific study and research concerning diet and health have ramped up. Dietary recommendations are quite different now from when I learned about "The Four Basic Food Groups" in elementary school. Not many people presently eat 7 – 10 servings of plant foods per day, but that is what nutrition experts are now recommending. Meat should be only a very small portion of a healthy diet if you choose to consume it at all. Water is the recommended beverage of choice for the health-conscious individual. Sugar and salt are toxins, and fat of all kinds should be very limited. Surprised?

In my search for better health, I had to essentially forget everything I thought I knew about nutrition, reprogram my mind, and learn how to feed my body all over again, and I'm so glad I did. Following this new plant-based lifestyle, the excess pounds melted away, physical problems disappeared, and I have more energy now than ever before. Believe me, the benefits in your own life will make it well worth the effort it takes to learn how to shop and cook for better health.

This scripture passage in Proverbs tells us that "the waywardness of the simple will kill them, and the complacency of fools will destroy them." With obesity and lifestyle diseases at an all-time high, we can no longer afford to "love our simple ways." Scientists are now telling us how important natural whole foods are to our health and longevity. You better listen! You can ignore the truth, but you cannot change it. The truth is a law. A law doesn't go away just because you choose to ignore it, or you don't agree with it. If you don't obey a law, then you will suffer the consequences.

Wisdom's truth is all around us, but we must be aware. Wisdom calls out to us, but we must listen. To choose to ignore wisdom is to choose to accept the consequences—in this case, the physical harm we do to our bodies by poor diet and lifestyle choices. Be a wise consumer—fill your shopping cart with better health!

* *Eat To Live: the Revolutionary Formula for Fast and Sustained Weight Loss*, by Joel Fuhrman M.D., Little, Brown, 2005, pp. 53 – 54.

BATTLE PLAN
SEVEN ACTION STEPS TOWARD WISE EATING

1. Eat 7 – 10 servings of vegetables and fruit every day.
2. Trade your white rice for organic brown rice – more nutrition and fiber, plus it tastes better!
3. Eat whole foods as close to their natural state as possible. For example, choose raw pineapple over canned, whole raw apples over applesauce.
4. Reduce salt consumption. Avoid white, free-flowing salt completely and choose an unprocessed, natural variety such as Gray Celtic Sea Salt or Pink Himalayan Salt instead.
5. Consume whole grains instead of processed. Simple Old Fashioned Rolled Oats or Steel Cut Oats, Millet, or Quinoa are better for you than any boxed breakfast cereal.
6. Eat minimal amounts of healthy plant fats from olives, avocados, coconuts, nuts, and seeds instead of animal fats that will only raise cholesterol, clog your arteries, and promote cell inflammation.
7. Use organic plant milk instead of dairy. There are many varieties (almond, rice, cashew, soy, oat, coconut, hemp...) and flavors so experiment until you discover one you like. I find almond milk to be tasty, creamy, and available in many grocery stores.

Day 7 - Father Knows Best

Job 28:20-28

> *...Where then does wisdom come from? Where does understanding dwell?*
> *It is hidden from the eyes of every living thing, concealed even from the birds of the air.*
> *Destruction and Death say, 'Only a rumor of it has reached our ears.'*
> *God understands the way to it and he alone knows where it dwells,*
> *for he views the ends of the earth and sees everything under the heavens.*
> *When he established the force of the wind and measured out the waters,*
> *when he made a decree for the rain and a path for the thunderstorm,*
> *then he looked at wisdom and appraised it; he confirmed it and tested it.*
> *And he said to man, "The fear of the Lord—that is wisdom, and to shun evil is understanding."*

When I first started on my search for better health, I looked everywhere for information and advice. I read all kinds of health and diet books. I read hundreds of magazine and newspaper articles and spent countless hours on the Internet seeking information that would not only help me to lose weight, but also conquer my physical problems. I was in my mid-forties and had come to realize that if I didn't change something I wasn't going to live to a ripe old age in vibrant health as planned. At that point some of my friends were starting to get desperately ill—a few had died. I watched helplessly as they endured torturous medical procedures and survived on a daily regimen of prescription drugs, going from one specialist to another only to be told that they needed yet another expensive medical test, treatment, or prescription, each with its own list of side effects or an extensive recovery period. I knew there had to be a better way! I prayed the Lord would show me.

I shuddered to think that this feeble premature end of life I was witnessing was God's ideal plan for his people. The second half of life should not be that painful and costly! When reading my Bible I noticed how the patriarchs in scripture died. Their deaths did not seem premature, prolonged, or painful. Instead, the norm was that they died "at a good old age, an old man and full of years." (Genesis 25:8, Genesis 35:28-29). They blessed their children, then peacefully climbed into bed and died. (Genesis 49:33)

Ah-hah! The answer to a long and healthy life must be found in the Bible, God's recorded history and guide for His children to follow here on earth. Until then I had been doing a lot of research in modern sources. With this revelation, I started to dig into God's Word for answers.

Job 28:20-28 says that Wisdom resides in God and His Word. The wisdom of this world, all the medical "breakthroughs" and health gurus' advice I had researched, is only "a rumor" of the wealth of knowledge and understanding—the hidden riches—to be found in God. What is a rumor? By definition, a rumor is "a perversion of the truth, a statement not based on reality." (Maybe that is why we keep hearing about new diets and health fads almost weekly).

In contrast, the wisdom in God's Word is truth. We can trust it because He has already studied, tested, and perfected it. Millions of research dollars, another double-blind study, and clinical trials are unnecessary. The wisdom of God is true and always works. It is a natural law. We don't have to wonder if God's way works—it does!

So, what is God's wisdom pertaining to health? Here is a snapshot of God's perfect plan for His creation (Please read these verses in the Bible for yourself):

Genesis 1:27 – God made man and woman with physical bodies to live in the physical world.

Genesis 1:29 – God told them to eat a plant-based diet to maintain their physical bodies in perfect health.

Genesis 2:15 – God told them to work in the garden because He knew that humans also need sunshine (vitamin D), fresh air, and physical labor to be physically fit, mentally alert, and content.

Following the wisdom of God, people lived illness-free with a lifespan of over 900 years until the time of the flood when meat was introduced into their diet (Genesis 6:3,7-8 and Genesis 9:2-3) and environmental changes occurred. Then man's lifespan rapidly declined. Did eating meat contribute to the decreased lifespan of man? Sarah died ten generations after Noah who lived to be 950, and she was only 127 years old. Just ten generations after Sarah, King David died between the ages of 70 – 80. That's a pretty dramatic drop in age!

Today scientists are beginning to affirm what God's Word revealed so long ago. Books like The Okinawa Diet Plan, by Bradley Wilcox, MD, MPH, D. Craig Wilcox, and Makoto Suzuki shed light on the importance of a lean body mass if you want to live a long and healthy life. Excess weight stresses the heart, blood vessels, and joints. It contributes to cancer risk, dementia, and macular degeneration, reducing not only length but also quality of life in later years.

A recent study in The Journal of the American Medical Association reported that overweight people who cut their daily calorie intake by 25% were more likely to have a lower core body temperature and normal fasting levels of insulin in their blood. Cutting calories just 15%, a 36-year study showed, produces a lower metabolic rate;

this means your body produces fewer free radicals, the root cause of degenerative disease. Cutting calories is easy to do if you take out the calorie- and fat-laden animal foods and replace them with whole plant foods.

It sounds so simple. It sounds so inexpensive. It sounds so easy. So why aren't we doing it? Why do Christians trust the rumor of wisdom found in the world's system instead of the wisdom of our Lord and Creator? The latest celebrity-endorsed fad diet is only a "rumor of wisdom." God's true wisdom endorses a whole-food, plant-based diet and physical exercise out in the sunshine and fresh air. Wisdom resides with God—in His Word. You can trust it! His original diet was and still is the healthiest way to eat. I guess Father still knows best!

BATTLE PLAN
DAD'S TEX-MEX BEANS

1 15 oz. can organic black beans, rinsed and drained

1 15 oz. can organic red kidney beans, rinsed and drained

1 15 oz can organic corn, rinsed and drained

½ medium red onion, chopped

2 stalks organic celery, chopped

¾ cup chunky salsa

2 tsp. ground cumin

Juice of 1 – 2 limes (to taste)

Salt (to taste), if desired

Cayenne pepper according to how spicy you like it

Mix all ingredients together in a large bowl at least one hour before serving to allow flavors to marinate. You could also make it the night before.

Refrigerate, and toss before serving.

Day 8 - The King is Watching

Daniel 1:8, 11-18, 20

But Daniel resolved not to defile himself with the royal food and wine, and he asked the chief official for permission not to defile himself this way. ... Daniel then said to the guard whom the chief official had appointed over Daniel, Hananaiah, Mishael, and Azariah, "Please test your servants for ten days: Give us nothing but vegetables to eat and water to drink. Then compare our appearance with that of the young men who eat the royal food, and treat your servants in accordance with what you see." So he agreed to this and tested them for ten days. At the end of the ten days they looked healthier and better nourished than any of the young men who ate the royal food. So the guard took away their choice food and the wine they were to drink and gave them vegetables instead. To these four young men God gave knowledge and understanding of all kinds of literature and learning. And Daniel could understand visions and dreams of all kinds. At the end of the time set by the king to bring them in, the chief official presented them to Nebuchadnezzar.... In every matter of wisdom and understanding about which the king questioned them, he found them ten times better than all the magicians and enchanters in his whole kingdom.

Daniel 2:48-49 – Then the king placed Daniel in a high position and lavished many gifts on him. He made him ruler over the entire province of Babylon and placed him in charge of all its wise men. Moreover, at Daniel's request the king appointed Shadrach, Meshach, and Abednego administrators over the province of Babylon, while Daniel himself remained at the royal court.

At the beginning of this story, we see a group of Hebrew boys, probably in their early teens, who were taken into exile by their Babylonian captors. These boys were specifically chosen because of their noble birth, exceptional physical appearance, and intelligence to be trained to serve in the conquering king's court. They were to undergo complete brainwashing, including being given new names and a complete change in diet to help them adjust and thrive in their new environment. As far as we can tell, they had it pretty good: comfortable accommodations, daily gourmet dining, and the best education available in the ancient world.

But one of these boys, Daniel, made a decision. Every important thing we do in life starts with a quality decision. Daniel "resolved (decided) not to defile himself with the king's rich food." Then he acted on that decision. A decision without action means nothing. Daniel asked for permission for him and his three friends to eat only vegetables and drink only water for ten days. This was not a test for Daniel and his friends. We can assume this was their normal diet up until this time, and the diet which had caused them to be judged physically and mentally superior in the first place. This ten-day testing period was to prove to the guard that a natural vegetarian diet wouldn't harm them. It is surprising to note that after only ten days on the king's diet, the other young men were visibly inferior to Daniel and his friends who were eating only whole plant foods and drinking clear, pure water. (Please note: it doesn't take long to observe physical changes after a positive dietary change).

From that time onward these four Hebrew young men were given only plant-based foods to eat and water to drink. Verse 5 tells us that the training period lasted three years, so we know this was their daily diet for at least three years, not the ten days we typically ascribe to Daniel's "fast." In reality, this vegetarian diet was not a fast at all; it was their normal lifestyle.

Daniel and his friends didn't conform to the king's orders even though that would have been the easy, comfortable, politically correct thing to do. I think they sensed that

God had put them in that place, at that time, to do something important for Him, and they needed to be at the top of their game to accomplish that task. They were willing to obey the Lord, stepping away from the crowd and doing what they knew was right. For us it is easy and comfortable to eat the Standard American Diet (SAD), which many consider to be the best diet in the world, but does that really please God? Is it beneficial for us?

In verse 17 we see that because they resisted the temptation to eat the king's rich food and stood strong in the face of worldly pressures and because they stepped away from the crowd and honored God in their bodies, God gave them knowledge, understanding, and wisdom, and to Daniel, the ability to interpret dreams. God is always looking for people who are faithful in the little things before He trusts them with larger responsibilities. Have you ever noticed that great men of God today didn't one day simply decide to stand up before a congregation and start preaching? Most have spent a long time before that public moment doing smaller jobs in the church such as teaching Sunday School classes or volunteering to help with Vacation Bible School. They humbly drive the church van, sweep floors, or stack chairs if that is what's needed. Many go to Bible College for years and then intern with an experienced pastor before the Lord will trust them with an entire congregation of His people. God is always looking for faithful servants. Are you one of them?

Daniel 2:48-49 describes the rewards the earthly king, Nebuchadnezzar, bestowed on these four brave young men. I don't believe the king would have even noticed them among the group of captives if they hadn't had the courage and conviction to be leaders and not followers from day one. They stepped away from the crowd, stood up for what they knew was right, and politely voiced their opinion. Their integrity and faithfulness made them different from the rest, and the king was watching.

Luke 16:10 tells us: "He that is faithful in that which is least is faithful also in much...." (KJB) Are you asking God for a ministry in his kingdom—a leadership role in His church? Maybe the place to start is with the little things like your diet and lifestyle habits. The King is watching!

BATTLE PLAN
DANIEL'S WINNING STRATEGY

- Be a leader, stand up for what you know is best for your body.
- Be brave enough to be different from the crowd.
- Be strong in your conviction to pursue a healthy lifestyle.
- Be faithful in the little things like diet and exercise.
- Be committed for the long term, not just for ten days.

Day 9 - Your Talent

Matthew 25:14-30

Again, it will be like a man going on a journey, who called his servants and entrusted his property to them. To one he gave five talents of money, to another two talents, and to another one talent, each according to his ability. Then he went on his journey. The man who had received the five talents went at once and put his money to work and gained five more. So also, the one with the two talents gained two more. But the man who had received the one talent went off, dug a hole in the ground and hid his master's money.

After a long time the master of those servants returned and settled accounts with them. The man who had received the five talents brought another five. "Master," he said, "you entrusted me with five talents. See, I have gained five more."

His master replied, "Well done, good and faithful servant! You have been faithful with a few things; I will put you in charge of many things. Come and share your master's happiness!"

The man with the two talents also came. "Master," he said, "you entrusted me with two talents; see I have gained two more."

His master replied, "Well done, good and faithful servant! You have been faithful with a few things; I will put you in charge of many things. Come and share your master's happiness."

Then the man who had received the one talent came. "Master," he said, "I knew that you are a hard man, harvesting where you have not sown and gathering where you have not scattered seed. So I

> was afraid and went and hid your talent in the ground. See, here is what belongs to you."
>
> His master replied, "You wicked, lazy servant! So you knew that I harvest where I have not sown and gather where I have not scattered seed? Well then, you should have put my money on deposit with the bankers, so that when I returned I would have received it back with interest.
>
> So take the talent from him and give it to the one who has the ten talents. For everyone who has will be given more, and he will have an abundance. Whoever does not have, even what he has will be taken from him. And throw that worthless servant outside, into the darkness, where there will be weeping and gnashing of teeth."

Have you ever wished you possessed the talents of another person? Have you ever envied someone else's ability or possessions; someone else's ministry? I confess; I have. We can all look around us and see other people who have more money, more creativity, more musical ability, more physical prowess, etc. than we have. Even though you may never be a billionaire or perform at The Metropolitan Opera House and even if you never win an Olympic Gold Medal, please do not be envious or compare yourself to the current "star of the month." Each person is accountable to God only for how we use our own talents.

There are many things in life that we may never have or do, but there is one "talent" which we all possess from the day we are born. Rich or poor, famous or obscure, we each possess the gift of a physical body, which the Lord has entrusted to our personal care.

Most of us come into this world in excellent physical condition. Barring birth defects, babies usually arrive healthy, active, and strong (at least their lungs are strong). What happens after birth, however, is influenced by many variables that can affect the human body in either good or bad ways. Continued good health does not happen by accident.

Diet is a crucial factor in maintaining health. Our bodies are composed of trillions of living cells. These living cells need living (raw) foods to nourish them and to build new healthy living cells as the physical body grows and develops. This is why God placed Adam and Eve in a garden in the first place. In the Garden, there was a constant abundant supply of luscious raw fruits and vegetables— the perfect foods to keep humans healthy and strong. Since the human body has not really changed since creation, doesn't it stand to reason that the perfect diet for modern humans hasn't changed from the original diet either? If you are not feeling healthy and strong, take a look at your diet. Does it resemble the original diet God planned for His people to eat?

If you are not sure you're eating healthfully, try keeping a food journal. For one full week don't change your diet at all, but write down everything you eat and drink. Not just at mealtimes, but for the entire 24-hour day simply jot down everything that goes into your mouth: every meal, every snack, every beverage, even every piece of chewing gum.

At the end of the week, honestly examine your 7-day food journal. What do you see there? Is there an apparent pattern to your eating habits? Statistics reveal that most Americans do not eat more than two servings of plant foods per day. Are you eating the seven to ten daily servings of vegetables and fruit required for optimal health? If not, then this is a good place to start. Don't count calories, fiber, fat percentages, or protein grams. All that will automatically balance out on a healthy vegetarian diet without you even having to think about it. Simply strive to consume seven to ten vegetables and fruits daily (more vegetables than fruit since many fruits are high in sugar).

To the 7 – 10 servings of vegetables and fruit, add several servings of whole grains, nuts, and legumes (peas, beans, lentils) to round out your healthy diet. This sounds like a lot of food, and it is. You can't possibly eat this way and continue to support the world's diet of animal products and junk food; there just isn't that much room in your stomach! But think about it... God didn't include these nutritionally void, fat- and calorie-rich foods in His original diet either. People thrived for more than the first one thousand years without any recorded incidence of disease on only what they planted and grew themselves. This could be a key to solving your health problems! A huge bonus is that when you are eating God's foods, the way he created them, you can't possibly be hungry or overeat because your diet is nutrient-rich, not calorie-dense. Many over-fed people today are starving because much of what they consume is processed fat and calories, so they overeat because their bodies are still craving the vitamins and minerals only found in real food.

Adam and Eve drank water. Do you? We're not talking about tap water, which contains far too many chemicals, but purified water that flushes toxins from your body as it hydrates your cells. It nourishes the lymph system and strengthens your immune system. The human body is composed of almost 60% water. The brain is 70% water, and the lungs are nearly 90% water. Add to that the fact that you are constantly losing water through perspiration, digestion, respiration, and cell repair even if you aren't doing any physical labor. Some of your fluid requirement can come through soups and freshly extracted vegetable or fruit juices, but it is impossible to have a healthy body if it isn't properly hydrated. Coffee, tea, and sodas are diuretics. They take water out of the body and do not provide proper hydration. The average person needs a minimum of eight, 8 oz. glasses of pure water each day, and even more if you are active, pregnant, or nursing.

A healthy body also needs sunshine for Vitamin D and physical exercise every day. Even a perfect diet will not make up for a sedentary lifestyle. It has been said that sitting is the new smoking. Muscles atrophy and flab increases even on thin people who don't exercise regularly. Remember, too, your heart is the most important muscle in your body, pumping blood to every part of the body 24 hours a day even while you are asleep. So, it is imperative to work your heart muscle through regular physical exercise if you want it to be strong. Your lymph system filters out bacteria and other foreign invaders to help you fight off disease; however, it has no heart muscle to pump the lymphatic fluid to where it is needed. The only circulation your lymph system has is what you create yourself by moving your body, so being active is essential for a healthy immune system. It's up to you.

You don't need to block out 2 hours per day for a gym workout if you just make a few modifications to your daily routine. Take a walk. Or better yet, walk the dog and you'll both get some exercise. (Have you ever noticed that overweight owners tend to have overweight pets?) Take the kids to the park and play with them—don't just sit on the bench looking at your cellphone or chatting with the other parents or grandparents. Plan to take the stairs instead of the elevator whenever possible. Park as far away from the store or office as you can; smile as you stride across the parking lot knowing that you are doing something wonderful for your body. Wear a pedometer and aim for 10,000 steps each day. Pump those arms, then do some wall push-ups (who needs weights). If you are addicted to TV, promise yourself that you will jog or march in place while you watch—at least during the commercials. Be creative and have fun thinking up new ways to squeeze physical exercise into your busy day.

Soon you will begin to see positive changes in your body. People will tell you how good you look, and you will feel great. Your clothes will fit better, or (and this is fun) you may even need to buy new clothes because the old ones are just too baggy! The best part is that you will be strong and healthy with enough energy to do whatever you want to do, or better yet, whatever God asks you to do.

The message of The Parable of the Talents is clear. God expects us to do the best we can for His kingdom with whatever He has entrusted to our care here on earth. Someday we will have to give an account of how we have handled the talents we've been given… even what we have done with the physical body He gave us. Do you want God to approve of the way you have cared for your body? Do you want Him to know that He can trust you right now with even more responsibilities in His Kingdom? Most of all, do you want to hear Him say, "Well done, good and faithful servant!"

BATTLE PLAN
SAMPLE FOOD JOURNAL PAGE*

BREAKFAST

LUNCH

DINNER

SNACKS

*Additional journal pages available at the end of the book.

Day 10 - Snakes Among Us

Numbers 21:4-9

They traveled from Mount Hor along the route to the Red Sea, to go around Edom. But the people grew impatient along the way; they spoke against God and against Moses, and said, "Why have you brought us up out of Egypt to die in the desert? There is no bread! There is no water! And we detest this miserable food!"

Then the Lord sent venomous snakes among them; they bit the people and many Israelites died. The people came to Moses and said, "We sinned when we spoke against the Lord and against you. Pray that the Lord will take the snakes away from us." So Moses prayed for the people.

The Lord said to Moses, "Make a snake and put it up on a pole; anyone who is bitten can look at it and live." So Moses made a bronze snake and put it up on a pole. Then when anyone was bitten by a snake and looked at the bronze snake, he lived

At the beginning of this story, as the children of Israel made their way through the wilderness, everyone was alive and well. Even in the middle of a desert, with no food or water, God's provision and protection were perfect. God provided manna which they gathered from the ground every morning. It was a perfect and versatile food that could be ground into flour, baked, or boiled. It only had to be gathered each day, and there was always enough. For forty years God's provision was sufficient to keep sickness and death out of the camp, and no one was hungry. But, instead of rejoicing in this divine health plan, the people started to complain about the things they lacked. They even found fault with God's perfect provision saying,"... we hate this miserable food!"

When the people rebelled against the Lord's provision, venomous snakes began to attack them. At first, I'm sure the Israelites didn't even notice as the snakes, camouflaged against the earth, slithered silently around the rocks and through the weeds until one by one the snakes started to viciously spring upon the unsuspecting complainers. As the children of Israel looked around, they were stunned to see dozens of snakes, hundreds of snakes, maybe more. One by one the people started to fall, victims of the poisonous intruders in their camp. The Bible tells us that "many Israelites died" from the venomous bites.

When the people realized what they had done and the severity of the consequences of their actions, they quickly repented (yet again) and begged Moses to pray for the Lord to remove the snakes from their camp. Does this remind you of modern Christians? We know that God's way is best. We trust Him in every area of our life...well almost. We know that we should be content with the perfect whole natural foods God has given to us to maintain health and wellness, but until we experience the consequences of our poor diets and lifestyle choices, we don't even notice (or care to see) that, like the slithering snakes in the Israelite camp, sickness and death are poised to attack.

Just like the children of Israel, we are quick to pray for healing when the snakes (sickness and disease) strike. We run to the altar, add our name to the prayer chain, ask the elders to anoint us with oil...does God answer? Did God answer Moses when he prayed for the Israelites to be healed?

God did answer their prayer, but not in the way they would have liked. God did not remove the snakes. The consequences of their sin remained, just as the results of a lifetime of poor health habits may produce lingering illness even after we pray. God told Moses to make a bronze snake and put it on a pole. This snake on a pole has become the emblem of modern medicine. Modern medicine says, "Look to me and you will live." Well, sometimes even all the pills and treatments doctors and hospitals have to offer are not enough to fight our modern diseases, many of which are known to be rooted in poor diet and lifestyle choices. We must do something ourselves to address the cause of our distress. You may survive without treating the cause, but what will be the quality of your life? How much better it is to be content with the natural whole plant foods (our manna) that God originally provided to keep us healthy and our immune systems strong than to rely on the healthcare system to "fix us."

God wants His people to be robust and to live a full and active life. If you are praying for healing, then it is imperative that you trust God and clean up your diet, too. We must maintain a thankful spirit for the matchless wisdom of God, who generously and perfectly supplies for our health and vitality instead of allowing the world's diet to invade our camp and make us sick. Don't merely rely on a bronze snake on a pole to rescue you. Trust God's natural foods to create and maintain your physical health.

BATTLE PLAN
CABBAGE WALDORF SALAD (FOR A CROWD)

In a very large bowl place:

1 head cabbage, shredded

1½ cup organic celery, chopped

1 cup dried cranberries or organic white raisins

2 organic apples, diced

15–18 pitted dates, chopped

1½ cup chopped walnuts or pecans

1–2 cups organic seedless grapes, optional

Dressing: Mix together equal amounts of freshly squeezed lemon juice and raw honey until well blended.

Pour dressing over all other ingredients, and toss to coat. Add more dressing if necessary. Chill until served.

Day 11 - The Secret

Psalm 92:12-15

The righteous will flourish like a palm tree, they will grow like a cedar of Lebanon; planted in the house of the Lord, they will flourish in the courts of our God. They will still bear fruit in old age, they will stay fresh and green, proclaiming, "The Lord is upright; He is my Rock, and there is no wickedness in Him.

We've heard it a million times: "I don't want to get old, but the alternative is so much worse." Yes, it all comes down to attitude. No one welcomes a new gray hair or rejoices to see laugh lines turn into permanent wrinkles on their face. As hard as we may try to cover up the visible signs of aging with hair color, cosmetics, and even surgery, time marches on. Sooner or later we all reach the age of seniority.

For years I taught craft classes at a senior citizens' center and also at a retirement village. One of the perks of working with these seniors was that I got to hear their life stories: the amazing experiences they'd had, the difficult times they'd overcome, their joys, tragedies, wisdom, and advice. Their stories proved that it isn't what happens in your life, it's what you do with what happens that makes all the difference. They taught me so much!

As I listened, I was able to identify those who had a strong Christian faith and those who did not. Some stories were so depressing—a litany of complaints, bitterly blaming others for their lot in life, full of despair and regrets. I spent a lot of time trying to get these depressed seniors to see the bright side of their life and circumstances... to simply smile for a change.

Conversely, seniors who had a strong faith in God, despite having endured horrendous tragedies during their lifetime, had an inner calm and a deep peace that was reflected in their words and in their very countenance. Their eyes twinkled as they told stories about growing up poor without the barest of what we would consider essentials. They would smile as they remembered a lost loved one or calmly shared how they had learned to cope after a life-changing accident or illness. They knew a secret I was just beginning to understand. Their faith was not shaken by their experiences; it actually grew because of the rough times they had lived through. Some of these seniors came to craft class in a wheelchair; some had hands so gnarled with arthritis that they couldn't make the simplest project, but they came with a smile "just to visit." These weekly visits were like therapy for us all. Even the most pessimistic of the group were buoyed by the good spirits and positive words of those who knew "the secret."

I remember one elderly maiden lady. She lived in the nursing home section of the retirement village. A strong Christian in her nineties with no immediate family, heart and kidneys failing, she spent her days in her room with only staff and the occasional volunteer visitor stopping in. She had served God all her life, but as she grew more feeble she began to feel useless in service to her Lord. Suddenly, she had an idea; she would quietly share her faith with everyone she spoke with! She started by quoting a different Bible verse each day to the nurse who helped her get dressed in the morning. She witnessed to the technician who came to service her television. Even when she received a wrong number on the telephone in her room, that conversation was not over until she asked the caller if they knew her Lord and Savior. This woman was excited to greet each new day because she had invented a vibrant ministry right there in her own room. Her mind was sharp and active because she was always seeking new and creative ways to bless others. She privately prayed for everyone with whom she came in contact. People felt better just being around her and soon began stopping in to visit just to get a dose of her good cheer.

Certainly, when you've lived long enough you will have dealt with some difficult circumstances, and maybe you haven't always made the best choices in life. Satan loves to remind you of your failures, inadequacies, and losses because his ultimate goal is to destroy you (John 10:10*). Those who know "the secret" (the real secret), know that you learn from your failure and then forget about that defeat. God does. He wants you to remember the lesson but forget the failure.

Your future starts now. God is your Rock, and there is no wickedness or condemnation in Him. Your relationship with God is NUMBER ONE. If you prioritize and nurture it every day, then you will flourish like a green tree and bear fruit even in old age. At the end of life, you can always tell who those people are—they are the ones who know "the secret!"

*John 10:10 – The thief comes only to steal and kill and destroy; I have come that they may have life, and have it to the full.

BATTLE PLAN
PRAYER OF SUBMISSION AND RELIANCE ON GOD

Dear Lord,

I come to you now as I am. I admit that I haven't always been perfect. I've done bad things, and bad things have been done to me. Thank you for loving me anyway.

Please, help me as I try to honor you in every area of my life, including my thoughts and my attitude. I promise to spend time with you, my Rock and my Healer, every day. Help me to seek your strength when I feel my resolve to cleanse my mind wavering.

Please help me to recognize and resist the enemy's attempts to steal, kill, and destroy my joy. I will not be robbed! Help me to recognize and reject toxic thoughts and emotions as they occur. I know these thoughts don't come from You.

Father, I want to live a long and fruitful life serving you. I want to honor and praise You all the days of my life. You are my Help, my Strength, and my Redeemer!

Amen.

Day 12 - The Stomach God

Philippians 3:18-19

...many live as enemies of the cross of Christ. Their destiny is destruction, their god is their stomach, and their glory is in their shame. Their mind is on earthly things.

As a young Christian, ecstatic that my sins were forgiven and I was a new creation in Christ, I could not help but share my new-found faith and freedom with everyone. In the course of my "witnessing," I would excitedly tell my friends, "I can do whatever I want because I'm not under the law; I'm under grace and Jesus will forgive me when I sin if I just ask Him." I loved the concept of grace—what a deal! I wondered why all my friends were not as excited by my testimony as I was. Could it be that besides my words they were also witnessing my actions, my day-to-day living? I'm sure I disappointed many who watched me for evidence of a changed life which, I'm sorry to say, was slow in coming. We Christians often use our freedom in Christ as permission to do whatever we want, secure in the knowledge that "the blood of Jesus cleanses us from all unrighteousness." We do have an intellectual grasp of the doctrine of grace, but how poorly we honor that reality in our daily lives.

As born-again believers, who have been given a second chance to do things better this time, our lives should reflect and honor our Savior in every way. Our lifestyle habits should not be exempt from a multi-faceted testimony we live out before the world. We are spirit, mind, and body, and our transformation should be evident in each of those areas so that even if we don't speak a word people will notice and ask what is different about us.

In Christian circles, gluttony seems to be the one acceptable vice. Overindulgence is chuckled about, promoted, and shared. If you've ever attended a church potluck dinner, you know what I mean. Heard any sermons on gluttony or healthy eating recently? Probably not, because overeating and eating the wrong foods are bad habits that most Christians share with one another and the world.

Is it any wonder then that Christians also share in the world's illnesses? Obesity, high cholesterol, high blood pressure, adult-onset diabetes, Alzheimer's, and even some cancers can all be traced to a high fat/high protein diet. In fact, researchers tell us that Christians, as a group, are even more overweight than the general population in North America.* Is this the testimony of the abundant life we want the world to see?

We don't intentionally desire to dishonor the cross by making our stomachs a controlling god in our life. Philippians 3:19 warns us that to do so leads to destruction. The gradual weight gain will take us down a path of physical degeneration and spiritual ineffectiveness we never intended to travel. We must not focus merely on earthly things, gratifying our fleshly desires with poor food choices. Satan loves to see Christians gorging on junk food. Even if you are one of those rare individuals who can eat anything and never gain a pound, you can still be physically malnourished and a prime candidate for degenerative illness. Satan knows that an overfed, tired, and sick Christian is too busy going from doctor to pharmacy to hospital, and praying for her own healing, to do much to save the lost or care for the needy of this world.

Earlier in Philippians 3 (v.16), the Word tells us to "live up to what we have already attained." Let's try to live up to God's ideal instead of sinking toward the world's junk-food diet. Strive to be a living testimony of God's saving grace in every area of life: spirit, mind, and body. The Savior, not your stomach, belongs on your heart's throne.

*Kenneth F. Ferraro, "Firm Believers? Religion, Body Weight, and Well-Being." Review of Religious Research," vol. 39, no. 3, 1998, p.224.

*https://www.foxnews.com/opinion/fat-in-church

BATTLE PLAN
SIMPLE "GREEN GOODNESS" SALAD DRESSING

1 ripe avocado (skin should be bronze and only slightly soft, not squishy)

1 garlic clove, peeled

1 lemon, juiced

Celtic sea salt to taste

Water (purified, distilled, or spring)

Optional: 1 tsp dried dill weed

Peel and pit the avocado and place it in a blender along with garlic, lemon juice, and seasoning. Add just enough water to cover. Blend until creamy. You may add more water until dressing reaches the desired consistency. Adjust seasonings as necessary.

Why buy bottled dressing when it's so easy to make your own fresh?

Day 13 - Food to Die For

Proverbs: 9:11, 17-18

For through me (wisdom) your days will be many and years will be added to your life. ...Stolen water is sweet; food eaten in secret is delicious! But little do they know that the dead are there, that her guests are in the depths of the grave.

When I started to seek answers for my own health problems, as a Christian I instinctively turned to the Bible, my handbook and guide for daily living. I began searching the scriptures to learn everything I could about God's perspective on health and healing. Why? Because the Bible says, "The fear of (reverence for) the Lord is wisdom" (Job 28: 28), and Proverbs 9:11 assures me that "through wisdom your days will be many and years will be added to your life." Wisdom about my health questions was exactly what I needed!

I am always humbled by the thought that God gave us the wisdom of the ages all written down in His inspired Word, the Holy Bible. Maybe it has been a while since you have opened your Bible. Maybe you've never even thought to ask God a specific question and then searched the scriptures to see what He has to say on the subject. I challenge you to try doing just that.

It is amazing to see that God has so much to say about what we should eat and how we should live to maintain total health. As I read, I realized again that God's living Word has as much to say to me, a twenty-first-century woman, as it did to a teenager two thousand years ago, and it will to a ninety-year-old senior citizen living in the future. God's Word is timeless! Some things that stood out as I studied were the ideals of discipline and integrity even in our eating habits. I had read Proverbs 9:17-18 before and traditionally thought of those verses as being pointed toward sexual temptation and sin. That symbolism is often taken for granted by those who read and teach these verses, so I did also.

However, the word "sex" is never mentioned in this passage. So, let's assume that the word "food" here literally does mean food, and read verses 17 and 18 in that light. As you read, do you get a mental picture of a bathrobed "someone" sneaking into a darkened kitchen after midnight, rummaging in the refrigerator for a late snack? Do you see someone quietly lifting the lid of the cookie jar as they glance over their shoulder, stuffing their pockets, and then gently replacing the lid so no one will hear? Maybe you see someone accepting delivery of a large "everything" pizza to be eaten alone where no one else can see? Do you see someone polishing off an entire carton of ice cream or a family-size bag of chips in front of the blue glow of the TV? Do you see... yourself?

Whom are we kidding? Even if no one else sees what we do in secret, our bodies know when we are feeding them too many calories or just plain junk food instead of the nutritious whole foods we need to stay healthy. And, guess what—our bodies tell on us! When our clothes no longer fit properly, when we're too poorly nourished to even fight off the common cold, when we have no energy to do the fun things we once enjoyed—everyone knows we didn't get that way by eating vegetables! The doctor knows, too. When he tells you that you need to lose weight and bring that cholesterol number or blood pressure reading down, or you will be a prime candidate for a heart attack...he knows! Scales and blood tests don't lie. You are not fooling anyone by gorging on junk food when you're alone. Your body will exhibit the evidence of your secret feasting, and the ultimate result of this lack of discipline will be premature death. Your doctor knows this, and the Bible warns us. So, stop lying to yourself.

A person of integrity does not lie to others or to herself. A person of integrity does not abuse her body with killer junk food. "Food eaten in secret" may be delicious, but is it worth dying for?

BATTLE PLAN
INNOCENT ICE CREAM

Here is a creamy, good-for-your-body treat you can eat without guilt!

Ingredients (per serving):
1 frozen banana
1 generous handful of frozen blueberries or strawberries

You can make this in a Champion Juicer or a food processor.

Using a Champion Juicer (with the blank instead of the juice screen): Simply feed pieces of frozen banana and frozen berries alternately through the juicer. What comes out will be yummy banana-berry "ice cream."

Using a food processor: Place broken pieces of frozen banana and frozen berries in the food processor, and blend until smooth. You may have to add a few tablespoons of plant milk to achieve ultimate creaminess using this method.

Enjoy!

Day 14 - Keep Your Eyes on the Prize

Jeremiah 32:31, 33-34

From the day it was built until now, this city has so aroused my anger and wrath that I must remove it from my sight. ...They turned their backs to me and not their faces; though I taught them again and again, they would not listen or respond to discipline. They set up their abominable idols in the house that bears my Name and defiled it.

Jeremiah 33:6 – Nevertheless, I will bring health and healing to it; I will heal my people and will let them enjoy abundant peace and security.

Have you noticed how modern-day awards are handed out to our children? The soccer coach no longer gives trophies to "The Most Valuable Player" or "The Player Who Scored the Most Goals." Today children receive trophies for "The Player with the Biggest Smile" or "The Player with the Best Attitude." When did things change? When did we start rewarding children for simply showing up and being nice?

I remember a time when kids wanted that trophy so badly that they were willing to devote every spare minute to practicing their sport. They were at practice every day even in rain and snow. When they weren't at practice, they kicked goals against the backyard fence. They tied a soccer ball on a rope around their waist and practiced their dribbling wherever they went. Their eyes were always on the prize. They even slept with their soccer ball. What were they dreaming about? Soccer! Why? Because they wanted to excel, to be the best, win the championship, and get that trophy!

This quest for a desired reward creates a disciplined lifestyle and is a living demonstration that hard work and daily practice do pay off. We want our kids to learn this lesson early, so we cheer their efforts in whatever sport they choose to participate in. Rarely does anyone succeed at any worthwhile endeavor without considerable diligence and persistence, including health. Do you want a healthy body? Do you care enough about your health to do whatever it takes to win that prize?

When the children of Israel ignored the Lord's instruction, brought idols into God's house, and worshipped them, God's anger was provoked. He promised in His Word to destroy that house that bears His name, and He sent the Babylonian invaders to do just that.

You are the temple of the Holy Spirit. When you set up idols of food, drink, or physical laziness, you are not honoring God in His temple; you are honoring the gods of appetite and sloth. When you ignore God's instructions for diet and lifestyle (Genesis 1:29, Genesis 2:15) just to gratify your own cravings, you set yourself up for the destruction of your body. Are you wondering what these worldly idols look like? They are anything you know to be unfit to maintain a healthy body, but you choose to bring them into your temple anyway: high fat, hormone and antibiotic-laced animal foods, fast foods, most prepackaged convenience foods, sugary or salty junk foods loaded with preservatives, and the nutritionally empty chemical concoctions we call soft drinks. What invaders will ultimately destroy your body temple? Excess weight, high cholesterol, physical disease, and finally an untimely and often painful death.

However, we serve a loving God. Just as He was willing to forgive Israel if they changed their ways, your Heavenly Father is anxious to forgive and reward everyone who makes the quality decision to turn from worldly idols and return to Him, the Author of Life. If you discipline yourself to eat His natural whole food, plant-based diet and drink the pure clean water God gave mankind in The Garden, if you daily engage in some type of physical exercise out in the sunshine, He will restore your path to physical health and healing where there was once destruction and disease. Your body is designed to heal, and it is amazing how quickly the human body responds to positive lifestyle changes. You will notice dramatic improvements in just a matter of weeks, but don't stop there! It's a total and forever lifestyle makeover—not a fad diet or a gym membership that expires.

Your Coach wants you to win this game, but He does not give the trophies of health and healing to His players simply because they're on "The Christian Team." These trophies can only be earned through a lifestyle that is focused and disciplined in every area. To do this you have to think about the way you are living. You must constantly ask yourself, "Does this food or activity contribute to, or detract from, the health of my body?" The answer should determine the choices you make.

Do you want that trophy? Then keep your eyes on the prize and do what it takes!

BATTLE PLAN
NO-BAKE GRANOLA BARS

4 cups organic old-fashioned rolled oats

1 cup raw sunflower seeds

½ cup chopped dates, organic raisins, or dried cranberries

¼ - ½ tsp sea salt

2 tsp. ground cinnamon

1/3 cup raw honey

½ cup tahini or cashew butter

½ cup chopped cashews

Juice of one orange

Combine all dry ingredients in a large bowl.

In another bowl, blend the cashew butter or tahini, raw honey, and orange juice. Pour this mixture over the dry ingredients and stir to mix well. (Mixture should hold together like a firm dough). If too crumbly add a little more orange juice.

Press dough into a lightly sprayed 8"x8" pan and refrigerate overnight. The next day cut into bars and wrap. The wrapped bars should be stored in an airtight container in the refrigerator (may also be frozen). If you like a crunchier texture you may dehydrate bars for 2-3 hours at low temperature. Cool before wrapping.

Day 15 - Don't Diet in a Donut Shop

James 1:14-15
but each one is tempted when, by his own evil desire, he is dragged away and enticed. Then, after desire has conceived, it gives birth to sin; and sin, when it is full-grown, gives birth to death.

When I was in college, one of my roommates worked in a donut shop, and at the end of each evening, she was permitted to take home as many unsold donuts as she wanted. As a result, we ate a lot of donuts back then! We were addicted to a daily fix of those deep-fat fried, sugary pastries. Years later, when I walk past a bakery that sweet aroma can still make my mouth water. When shopping for groceries, it's all I can do to pass through the bakery department without stopping to gaze at the glass case displaying dozens of plump fresh donuts—some filled with fruit or cream, some iced, glazed, or dipped in colored sprinkles.

Sigh...

Even as I peruse those donuts I ask myself, "What in the world are you doing here? Why tempt yourself?" I now know that donuts are bad for me. I know they are fried in oil, full of fat, calories, and processed sugar. I know they have absolutely no nutritional value and are loaded with cholesterol. I know all that sugar will depress my immune system, lowering my resistance to illness. I also know that donuts are one of my deep-rooted weaknesses, a habit I have worked hard to conquer. So, WHY am I drooling in front of the donut case?

I confess that I allow myself to be lured by this temptation because of my own evil desire. A donut in the eyes of a food addict can be just as seductive as a cocktail to an alcoholic or a needle to a drug addict. Just because donuts are sold in the supermarket doesn't make them safe or acceptable for consumption. You know the damage they do to your body. The same can be said for potato chips, bacon, cheeseburgers, candy bars, ice cream—whatever your fixation happens to be.

If you allow yourself to be in an area of temptation, you will eventually surrender to its enticement. Let's label that surrender exactly what it is: S-I-N. If you know that something is wrong, no matter what that "something" is, and you do it anyway, then you are sinning. Yes, let's be painfully honest: this even applies to our food choices.

James tells us that sin, when it is full-grown, gives birth to death. It can be a spiritual death where you no longer hear or even care about the Holy Spirit's conviction concerning the choices you make. In the case of diet, it can also be a literal physical death, where you actually eat yourself into a state of sickness or even an early grave—something many who consume the Standard American Diet (SAD) are doing every day. "Death by fork" should be written on many death certificates.

You know that you should be eating a healthy diet composed mainly of fresh, natural fruits, vegetables, whole grains, legumes, nuts, and seeds as close to the way God designed them as possible. You know that white flour, sugar, and animal products are unhealthy, so why put yourself where you will be tempted by these? As Christians, when we label the harmful objects of our desire S-I-N it is much easier to reject them. So, do your best to identify sin as soon as you recognize the desire. And please, don't try to diet in a donut shop—it just doesn't work!

BATTLE PLAN
COCONUTTY "DONUT HOLES"

These are gluten-free and a healthier way to occasionally satisfy your sweet tooth.

2 cups almonds or pecans (soaked overnight and drained)

1½ cups chopped dried pineapple and/or dates

1 tsp. vanilla

4 Tbs. dried unsweetened shredded coconut

Honey or maple syrup (a little to taste if desired)

Process nuts and fruit in a food processor using the S-blade. Add coconut and sweetener a little at a time. (Stop to scrape bowl several times). When mixture holds together and forms a dough, roll small amounts of dough into donut hole-size balls, and roll each ball in additional coconut. Store in an airtight container in the refrigerator.

Day 16 - Plan Your Way Out

1 Corinthians 10:13

No temptation has seized you except what is common to man. And God is faithful; He will not let you be tempted beyond what you can bear. But when you are tempted, He will also provide a way out so that you can stand up under it.

As Christians, we like to proclaim, "Greater is He that is in me than he that is in the world." Then we roll over and play the victim at an all-you-can-eat buffet. If God is faithful and we are more than conquerors, then what is going on here, temptation or addiction?

I hesitate to validate the term "food addiction" or "food addict," terms which allow some people to abdicate their own responsibility and God's willingness to help them bring their food cravings under control. God will not allow us to be tempted beyond what we can bear. So why do we allow that temptation to conquer us rather than standing firm, fighting back, and with God's help win the battle with our own flesh?

God's Word says (and God doesn't lie) that He will provide a way out so that you won't succumb to temptation. With just a little thought and a moment of rational inner dialogue with yourself, you should be able to design a plan to cope with any dietary temptation you are facing. The Lord will help you if you ask Him, but you must ask Him, and you must be willing to follow through on the plan once He reveals it to you.

For example, if food really is a struggle for you then maybe you shouldn't be at an all-you-can-eat buffet in the first place. (Hmmm-m-m, there's a thought.) Are you strong enough to pass up the barbequed spareribs, fried chicken, and ooey-gooey sweet desserts and instead create a satisfying meal at the salad bar? Be adventurous and try some new things on your salad; you might find something brand new to love. Have you ever tried baby corn, edamame, red beets, nuts, seeds, or dried fruit on a salad? (A word of caution: just because it's on the salad bar doesn't mean it belongs on a salad. Cottage cheese and creamy macaroni are not vegetables and do not belong on a salad bar or on your plate!) Can you be thankful for the healthy fresh foods you know you should be eating and not feel deprived passing up the tempting, processed rich foods on display? If you don't yet feel strong enough to do this, then please stay away from the buffets! As you can see there are at least two "ways out" provided for you here, but you must follow through with one of them.

How about coffee break time at work? Are there soda and candy machines in the break room? Donuts? Is it always someone's birthday, and there is leftover cake or open boxes of chocolates to share? If you know what to expect, then plan for it. What is your "way out"? You could keep a stash of healthy snacks in your desk drawer. Vegetables and fruit are nutrient-dense foods compared to sugary baked goods which are not simply empty calories but are also immune system suppressants. Who needs that? Plan to bring healthy snacks to work with you and keep a supply there at all times. A handful of raw almonds or walnuts will provide excellent plant-based protein and will help to keep you feeling full all afternoon. Whole-grain crackers with natural organic nut butter (just a few) is a satisfying snack. Quench sugar cravings with fresh juicy fruit. To avoid caffeine in the ever-present office coffeepot, you can keep a selection of herbal teas at your desk to sip with your healthy snack. And don't forget to pack your own bottle of purified water to drink throughout the day. If you design a plan for success, you will be able to indulge your cravings with healthy food choices, and you won't feel deprived during break time. You will avoid hunger pangs and be much more alert and energized than you would be if you had given in to the donut and coffee temptation.

When I first decided to change my eating habits I always carried a small plastic bag filled with dried fruit and nuts in my pocket and an apple plus a water bottle in the car. During this lifestyle change-over, I felt like I was always hungry. On many occasions those little snacks that I had the forethought to pack saved me from making a huge dietary fumble. However, once my body adjusted to a healthy diet, and became well-nourished, those cravings went away. Today I rarely snack between meals; I simply don't get hungry as I used to. This didn't happen all at once. It took 60 – 90 days of consistently eating healthy plant foods for me to be completely comfortable with this new and improved lifestyle. When you eat a nutrient-dense variety of foods, your body isn't on a constant search for the nutrition it needs. Overeating is not a problem. On a plant-based diet, your body will sense that it is well nourished and will naturally crave less food; unwanted pounds will fall away, and you will be much healthier in every respect. Today I can eat a nice big salad for lunch and be totally satisfied until supper time.

One thing that is never optional is water. Remember to drink purified or spring water between meals. Often thirst comes disguised as hunger, and I have noticed that if I drink 12 ounces of fresh water, then wait 10 minutes, I no longer feel hungry. Besides that, water is essential for the health and maintenance of every cell in your body. You can't live in health without being properly hydrated. It is also important to drink most of the water you consume between meals so that it doesn't dilute your digestive enzymes and interfere with your body's ability to process the meal.

You can do this. You are not the first person to be tempted by food (Adam and Eve were), but you can't allow these temptations to control you. God is faithful to provide a way out of temptation's grasp, but you must walk in that way. Don't close your eyes to His leading. Don't block your ears to His voice. That little whisper you hear telling you to not give in to your flesh, the tug you feel leading you away from the dessert table—that's God! He's showing you the way out! Trust Him. Follow Him ...away from temptation and into a healthier life.

BATTLE PLAN
BASIC HUMMUS

Hummus is a great staple in a plant-based diet. Because it is so easy and economical to make at home (or you can always buy it for 3 – 4 times the cost of homemade) I always have some in the refrigerator to use as a dip for raw vegetables and whole grain crackers or to spread on a veggie wrap. Here is a basic recipe, but you can add other optional ingredients such as roasted red pepper, cooked spinach, artichoke hearts, or black olives to change the flavor and color.

1 15 oz. can chickpeas, rinsed and drained

2 Tbs. tahini (sesame seed butter)

1 clove garlic

1 Tbs. fresh lemon juice

Sea salt to taste

Place all ingredients in a food processor or blender and blend to puree. Stop to scrape sides of bowl occasionally. Add optional ingredients when blending if desired. Add a little water, 1 tsp. at a time, if necessary. (Mixture does not have to be perfectly smooth). Refrigerate and serve cold.

Day 17 - Bless the Beasts

Exodus 23:5, 11-12

If you see the donkey of someone who hates you fallen down under its load, do not leave it there; be sure you help him with it....but during the seventh year let the land lie unplowed and unused. Then the poor among your people may get food from it, and the wild animals may eat what they leave. Do the same with your vineyard and your olive grove. Six days do your work, but on the seventh day do not work, so that your ox and your donkey may rest...

Long before animal rights became an issue God was expressing His concern for all His creatures. Although only humans are made in the image of God, that does not mean animals are expendable, without emotion, or unimportant in the eyes of God. Because you and I are made in the image of God, we should act as He would and not abuse His creatures. Jesus said, "Are not five sparrows sold for two pennies? Yet not one of them is forgotten by God." (Luke 12:6).

God loves all His animals. Do you think He approves of the daily suffering they endure in modern factory farms, where they are forced to live in filthy, cramped conditions and are subjected to unnatural diets and massive amounts of drugs during their short miserable lives just to increase profits? He is not pleased by the cruel slaughter of thousands of His animals every day just to satisfy the culture's gluttonous desire for animal flesh. God never intended for man, His highest creation, the one to whom He gave dominion over all the earth, to so devalue and inflict so much pain on the innocent animals we were supposed to take care of.

As a person of conscience, as one who has the Holy Spirit living in me, I cannot participate in and perpetuate the barbaric practices of the animal industry. If you would like to learn more about this topic, then I urge you to check out these resources: www.peta.org and www.tribeofheart.org. Watch some of the videos on those websites. It will be an eye-opening experience. Most Americans don't know anything about the unnecessary torture these animals endure just to feed our lust for their flesh. This is why the few times these horrors were given any media exposure those facilities were immediately shut down, and the people responsible were prosecuted. Still, animal factory farming is a huge government-protected business in our economy, and good people turn a blind eye. Just because we don't want to look at it doesn't mean it isn't happening. The horror continues.

Personally, I want to practice the art of "gentle living" in all areas of my life. I don't want any animal to suffer these barbaric abuses because of the food choices I make. Learning about the inhumane treatment of the animals we consume cemented in my mind the decision to listen to my conscience and eat a healthy cruelty-free diet. No animal needs to die for my dinner. Eating a plant-based diet is very easy to do now that many grocery stores, as well as health food stores, carry a vegetarian substitute for any animal product you desire. Today you can choose from several different brands of veggie burgers, veggie cheese, and every variety of "milk" under the sun (rice, soy, coconut, almond, cashew, hemp, oat, etc.). I have experimented and discovered many delicious vegetarian recipes my family loves, so eating this way is not difficult—it's just different from the way we used to eat.

The next time you go grocery shopping try some of the vegetarian options available. You may find that you like them! Plant-based substitutes for foods you already eat taste similar, but with lower fat, calories, and no cholesterol (only animal foods contain cholesterol). Your body will thank you. Why would anyone choose to eat a hamburger when you can have that taste and texture in a veggie burger with no bad health effects and no animal torture and death involved? It's a no-brainer! Also, if you are concerned about the environment, global warming, or the conservation of resources, then please understand that a plant-based lifestyle is the single most important thing you can do for the planet. It takes twelve times as much grain to feed a single cow as it does to feed a human. Think of that figure in terms of land resources, water resources, and energy resources all being depleted because Americans insist on eating animals. What a wasteful legacy for our children! Please realize we don't have a corn shortage because it is being made into cornflakes or ethanol. Shortages and high prices are the direct results of feeding most of our grain crops to animals! How many more starving people in the world could we feed instead?

We hear a lot about certain strains of bacteria and viruses becoming antibiotic-resistant. This isn't only because of the doctor prescribed antibiotics being consumed by people for their own medical treatment. Residue of the mass quantities of antibiotics fed to commercially raised animals ends up in our food chain, in the meat and eggs you consume, and in the milk you drink. If you eat animal foods, then you are ingesting antibiotics even if you don't have a prescription for them.

You cannot control the world's economy or change the "all American hot dog and apple pie" image of our country, but you can decide how you feed your own body. You can make conscious decisions when you grocery shop and when you eat out to not support the cruel wholesale slaughter of animals and the destruction of your planet. You can do something! Every time you drink almond milk instead of cow's milk or eat a vegetable stir-fry instead of steak or chicken, then you are doing something positive for yourself and for the world you live in. Why not?

In Genesis 1:28, God gave man dominion over all the world and the animals in it. He put us in charge of His entire creation. Let's be honorable managers and use this position of authority to be wise and loving caretakers instead of cruel and selfish tyrants. Our Heavenly Father entrusted us with a huge responsibility; let's not disappoint Him.

BATTLE PLAN
GRILLED NO-BEEF BURGER

4 large Portabella mushroom caps, washed and stems trimmed short

1/3 cup olive oil

2 – 3 Tbs. balsamic vinegar

1 tsp. dried basil

Salt and pepper to taste

In a small bowl whisk together olive oil, vinegar, and basil. Brush mixture liberally over mushrooms (both sides) and allow to marinate at least 30 minutes.

Sprinkle with salt and pepper if desired. Place foil on grill and spray to prevent sticking. Grill mushrooms several minutes on each side.

Serve on toasted whole-grain rolls with a slice of veggie cheese and your favorite burger toppings (Grilled onions and peppers are delicious on top).

You don't have to throw away your grill – enjoy the picnic!

Day 18 - Your Well

Proverbs 4:23
Above all else, guard your heart, for it is the wellspring of life.

Think of your heart as a well, "the wellspring of life." Every well depends on a strong efficient pump to deliver its contents. Without a good pump, the well is useless. Good wells are unpolluted and healthy. The water coming from them is crystal clear and clean. A healthy well produces all the pure water you need for cleansing and refreshment.

On the other hand, a contaminated well produces foul discolored water full of toxins you would rather avoid. When you notice that your drinking water has a "funny odor" or isn't clear, you instinctively refuse to drink it. The cells of your bodies, however, do not have that choice; the only cleansing, refreshing option your cells have is the blood pumped by your one-and-only heart through the arteries, veins, and capillaries that feed every thirsty cell. Weak or strong, clean or polluted, this is your cells' only option.

This verse concerning the heart has a clear spiritual as well as a physical application. The spiritual pertains to what affects your state of mind, feelings, and emotions. Anger, hatred, worry, and bitterness are examples of destructive emotions that contribute to broken relationships, isolation, and depression if they are allowed to fester and grow. These heart issues pollute your well and need to be dealt with and corrected now if you wish to pursue any measure of physical and mental health. These emotions are spiritual corrosives, and let's be honest, they are SINS. If indulged, these sins can mature into idols in your heart and mind.

Although you may be able to hide these idols from the rest of the world behind a great big Christian smile, you can't fool your own body. Inside, the emotional turmoil of anger, hurt, hatred, or grudges takes an extremely unhealthy toll on your entire body, not just your mind. Scientists tell us that the burden of mental anxiety has a very negative effect on the human body's ability to resist sickness and disease.* So, if you are in a constant state of emotional agitation, you are more likely to get sick; and if you are already sick, unresolved emotional stress could hinder your efforts to recover.

We all know that we need to "guard our hearts" physically. This is our motivation to work out at the gym, watch our weight, monitor our blood pressure, and regularly have our cholesterol levels checked. Our doctor tries to hold us accountable in this area because he realizes that you must maintain a healthy heart to avoid serious medical problems. He also knows that a healthy heart doesn't just happen!

From about the age of thirty, your body is no longer growing; it is aging. If you don't foster an environment of heart health through diet, exercise, and emotional well-being your heart, the most important and constantly working muscle within your body, will get weak and inefficient at pumping blood to the more than thirty trillion cells that depend on it for nourishment and regeneration. When these cells don't have the support of a healthy heart, they can't do their jobs and disease happens. ("Disease" definition: dis-ease; out of ease; out of order…in trouble!)

As the only caretaker of your well, it is up to you to maintain a strong healthy pump (heart). It is the only pump you have; there is no backup system for this well. In addition, you must not pour toxins or dirt into your well. You must not sabotage your well by smoking or ingesting any harmful substances. You must not eat overly processed, chemical-laden non-foods. ("Non-food" definition: something that is disguised as food, but is actually devoid of nourishment; i.e. just about anything that comes in a colorful box or a cellophane wrapper.) You must identify canned and bottled juices, sodas, and sports drinks as the chemical cocktails they are and choose to drink pure water instead. The fewer ingredients listed on any package, the better.

Finally, you must avoid artery-clogging, calorie-dense animal fats of all kinds. Choosing foods as close to the garden as possible (fresh, organic fruits and vegetables) will help your heart stay healthy and strong. If your veins and arteries are blocked by fat (atherosclerosis), if the blood supply is inferior due to poor diet, if your body is under the stress of negative emotions, then you can't expect to maintain and rebuild healthy cells anywhere in your body.

As you pursue a nutritious plant-based diet, begin to practice kindness, forgiveness, and trust in God; then you will relieve your heart of tremendous emotional strain. Can you see that your heart really is "the wellspring of life"? Your heart and circulatory system need all the help you can give to repair, fight disease, and nourish every cell in your body. You are purifying your well if you "guard your heart."

*None of These Diseases, by Dr. S.I. McMillen, Fleming H. Revell, 1993, pp. 57 - 67

BATTLE PLAN
HEART-HEALTHY RICE AND BEANS

Start with a pot of cooked or canned beans (kidney, navy, black, pinto...use any combination you like), rinsed and drained.

Put beans into a large pot and add any amount of rice you desire with twice as much water plus an extra 2 cups of water. Add salt to taste if desired. Stir together and heat to boiling. Lower heat and simmer. Total cooking time will vary depending on which type of rice you use, so follow package directions.

While rice cooks prepare 3 – 4 cups of finely chopped vegetables (onion, garlic, green and red bell pepper, celery, and carrot are a colorful combination). Add vegetables to the rice and bean mixture about 10 minutes before rice is done cooking, being careful to adjust heat to maintain cooking temperature. You want the vegetables to be crisp-tender, not overdone at the end of cooking time.

Taste and season to your liking with Bragg's Liquid Amino Acids or Herbamare and any additional spices you desire. I like turmeric for color and cilantro. Another variation: cumin and chili powder are also good with optional cayenne pepper for those who like it spicy.

Heart-Healthy Rice and Beans may be served as a main dish, a side dish, or in a tortilla wrap with veggie cheese, lettuce, tomato, guacamole, and salsa.

Day 19 - The Choice is Yours

Psalm 78:18, 29-31

They willfully put God to the test by demanding the food they craved. ...They ate till they had more than enough, for He had given them what they craved. But before they turned away from the food they craved, even while it was still in their mouths, God's anger rose against them; He put to death the sturdiest among them, cutting down the young men of Israel.

The array of food choices available to us today is mind-boggling. Our supermarkets are as big as department stores! We are constantly surrounded by a smorgasbord of enticing options, and sometimes we forget that everything available for us to consume is not always nourishing. Some things may not even be recognized by our bodies as food, and our bodies do not know how to process those things. This condition leads to toxic build-up and illness. Inferior, nutritionally empty "food" produces excess stored fat in our cells, clogged arteries, and chemical imbalances such as Type II Diabetes. Only the world's diet causes these dire consequences. God's diet does not. The whole foods our loving Father created for our sustenance in the beginning were designed to promote optimum health in the human body, not disease and decay.

Psalm 78 relates the ancient story of how the Israelites, wandering in the wilderness for forty years, complained about the manna that the Lord God caused to fall on the ground every morning for them to gather and eat that day. Manna was a perfect food; always delivered fresh, and it could be prepared in many ways. They didn't have to buy, plant, or cultivate it; it just appeared. This manna was such a unique and complete food that the Israelites didn't even know what to call it. "Manna" literally means "what is it?" It could be baked, boiled, or eaten fresh. "It was like coriander seed and tasted like wafers made with honey" (Exodus 16:31). This pure and matchless food is what God graciously supplied for their nourishment; it required no expense or labor on their part other than to gather it fresh every morning.

Despite God's miraculous provision for their dietary needs, and even though they were all well-fed and healthy on God's diet, the Israelites were not content. They missed the rich foods they had enjoyed in Egypt and demanded meat to eat (See Numbers 11:4-34). Because God never forces His will on anyone, He gave them exactly what they were craving and supplied an abundance of meat, swarms of quail, which they greedily devoured. The consequence was physical illness and their demise.

Does this sound at all similar to what we experience eating the Standard American Diet? God has graciously given us every delicious and nutritious plant food His earth produces, but that is not good enough for us. We crave the rich foods, many of which man has so chemically altered that our bodies are destroyed just trying to process them. God's perfect will is for us to follow the original whole food plant-based diet He designed to enable His people to walk in health and vitality. We are missing God's best for our health if we don't choose His superior natural foods over the world's empty imitations.

God wants us to eat fresh, brightly colored, living vegetables, fruits, legumes, nuts, whole grains, and seeds. That was His first diet for mankind, and it is still the healthiest. Animal foods are dead, inferior substitutes, devoid of fiber, and high in fat, calories, and cholesterol.

To make matters even worse, to increase production and profits, modern factory farm animals spend their short miserable lives crammed into tiny pens or cages where they can't even turn around, are pumped with hormones and antibiotics, and stuffed with chemically altered feed, which sometimes contains other dead animal parts. Because we know these contaminants are so bad for us, many consumers live in denial, unwilling to face the truth about the chemicals or cruelty in animal factory farming. We don't want either in our food supply, so why do we perpetuate this system? Are we that afraid of change? Unwilling to change? Are we such creatures of habit, or are we just plain lazy? Individually, we may not be able to transform the practices of global factory farming, but we CAN transform our own diets and in so doing collectively make an economic statement to the industry.

In addition, there are the many artificially colored, flavor-enhanced, sugar-coated or overly-salted, partially hydrogenated snacks and breakfast foods in slick colorful packages lining our grocery store shelves, seducing us to overload our bodies with empty calories. It all looks good, but we must remember that all these perversions of the natural whole foods God created attack our immune systems causing eventual physical stress, illness, and even death. As you read the list of ingredients on a box of cereal or package of snacks remember: the longer the list of ingredients the more perverted…I mean processed…it is. Man cannot improve on God's perfect foods.

Why then, you wonder, are all these food choices available to us if God doesn't want us to partake? God always allows us to make our own choices in life because He has made us creatures of free will, to ultimately and ideally choose Him and His ways. He will not stop us if we insist on "having what we crave." As in any area of life, however, we will suffer the consequences for any harmful choices we make. If it helps, think of it this way. When you are confronted with food options: You are not choosing between this food and that food; you are choosing between health and illness, between life and death.
Be wise—CHOOSE LIFE!

BATTLE PLAN
TIPS FOR HEALTHY EATING WHEN DINING OUT

The menu looks disappointing... what can I eat in this restaurant?

We all face this dilemma at some point when dining out, but I have discovered a few tricks to maintain a healthy diet even if there isn't a single vegetarian entrée on the menu:

- First of all, look at the soup, salad, and appetizer sections of the menu. You may find something suitable there. Many times, appetizers are meant for sharing (meaning huge), so one appetizer could easily be your whole dinner. One of our local restaurants has a delicious Hummus Platter appetizer (platter of fresh romaine lettuce generously topped with homemade roasted red pepper hummus and garnished with sliced tomatoes and warm toasted pita bread) that I adore. It is meant for four people to share as an appetizer, but I always order it for my entrée when we eat there, and it is more than enough.

- Look at the side dishes. You can certainly put together a satisfying meal of 3 – 4 vegetarian sides (not French fries, macaroni salad, and onion rings!) and a salad. Keep it simple and be creative.

- Sometimes you can find a great vegetarian pasta dish already on the menu, but if you can't then look at the options that are available and don't be afraid to ask if a dish you want could be prepared minus the meat and/or cheese. Most restaurants are happy to comply.

- If one entree comes with broccoli and another comes with mushrooms and peas, then ask your server if you could please have pasta or a baked potato topped with broccoli, mushrooms, and peas (because you know they already have those ingredients in house). Restaurants teach their staff that a satisfied customer will be a returning customer and will tell their friends. I request these little alterations to my order all the time and usually find the kitchen staff ready and willing to please.

- Finally, if all else fails just ask the chef if he can prepare a special meal that meets your dietary requirements. Some of the most beautiful and delicious restaurant meals we have enjoyed were the result of simply making that request. Many chefs welcome the challenge. You won't know if you don't ask.

So please don't be intimidated by menus or refuse to go out to eat because you're afraid you won't find anything on the menu to suit your new healthy lifestyle. Meet your friends for dinner! Enjoy their company, and don't stress out about what to eat. In the whole scheme of life, it is, after all, just one meal. You don't have to live like a hermit to eat healthily! You just have to be creative and enjoy the journey... To life!

Day 20 - Confession of Transgression

Psalm 32:1-5

Blessed is he whose transgressions are forgiven, whose sins are covered. Blessed is the man whose sin the Lord does not count against him and in whose spirit is no deceit. When I kept silent my bones wasted away through my groaning all day long. For day and night your hand was heavy upon me; my strength was sapped as in the heat of summer. Then I acknowledged my sin to you and did not cover up my iniquity. I said, "I will confess my transgressions to the Lord" – and you forgave the guilt of my sin.

"Mom, I did something really bad, and I'm sorry. I did it three weeks ago, and it's been bothering me ever since then, so I have to tell you about it." At ten years old, Aaron was not the type of child to have a heart-to-heart discussion with me about anything. He was the child who skipped walking down the last five steps, preferring to jump and crash land with a house rattling boom at the bottom every morning as he joined us for breakfast. Normally, he ran in and out of the house with a trail of little boys behind him, eating everything in their path and teasing little sisters along the way. Looking at his hunched shoulders and half-lowered head as he glanced up to gauge my reaction to the beginning of his confession, I knew that this was serious and I'd better sit down and listen right now. I sighed, wondering what he possibly could have done.

Giving him my full attention, I asked Aaron to explain. As the story unfolded, I learned that Aaron had carved a little hole in his closet wall so he could talk to his sister as she sat in her closet in the next room. (Whew, not as serious as the possibilities I was imagining just moments before!) Whispered conversations, secret messages written on notebook paper, rolled up, and slipped through that hole in the wall had been fun until his conscience kicked in. Then he started to worry night and day that the damage to his wall would be discovered; how would he explain? (I should mention that this hole was in a brand new wall in a brand new house we had just built – there was no way it wouldn't eventually be noticed and no way he could blame someone else). Instead of being fun, that hole became a scar—a constant reminder of the damage he had caused. He saw his transgression every day, and the burden grew heavier and heavier until he couldn't bear it any longer.

Aaron was relieved to have that confession off his chest, and although there were consequences (Dad showed him how to repair and repaint the wall himself the following Saturday), he learned that telling the truth when you mess up is always best, paying the price is easier than carrying the burden, and Mom and Dad love you no matter what you've done. Confession truly is good for the spirit!

King David learned about the effects of unconfessed sin in his own life when he tried to cover his sin of adultery with Bathsheba by having her husband, Uriah, killed in battle (2 Samuel:11). David soon realized that he couldn't hide his sin from others, and he couldn't ignore the shame he felt. The guilt of his sins not only caused him mental anguish but physical illness in his body. He moaned in feverish pain. It was so bad that he couldn't even eat. He was wasting away to skin and bones.

Trying to live each day under the burden of unconfessed sin puts tremendous stress on your body. Stress is an enormous contributor to heart attacks, not only causing arteries to constrict, but scientific studies show that it also makes the blood more likely to clot.* In addition, emotional stress is a factor in many other disabling conditions such as arthritis, digestive ailments, headaches, nervous tension, depression, and insomnia to name a few.

If you are trying to carry the burden of unconfessed sin by yourself, talk to your Heavenly Father about it. Trying to handle the guilt alone will only wear you out emotionally and physically. Don't worry, there is nothing you could tell God that He hasn't heard before, and the good news is that He loves you anyway. No matter what you have to say, He already knows all about it. God doesn't need to hear it, but you do need to tell it. There may be consequences to pay to make things right again, but they won't be as heavy as that burdened conscience you've been carrying.

He is waiting NOW with arms wide open for you to make the first move. Run into those arms! Tell Him the whole story and let Him comfort you. It will be such a relief to lay that heavy burden down. Do it NOW. Confessed sin leads us to forgiveness and salvation. It is the beginning of a blessed life, a healthy life.

*None of These Diseases, S.I. McMillan, Fleming H. Revell, 1993, pgs. 92-94.

BATTLE PLAN
PRAYER OF CONFESSION*

Father, I've blown it. I recognize and confess that there is sin in my life, and I am suffering because of it. I acknowledge my guilt. I renounce and repent of the sin of

_____. I'm sorry that I was weak and selfishly chose to do things my own way instead of ignoring what I know is right in your sight. I humbly ask your forgiveness, Lord. I love you, and I am grateful that even though I don't deserve it, you love me enough to cover my sin with your own blood sacrifice. Please give me the strength to make things right and to recover from my disobedience. With your help, from now on I will try to honor you in every area of my life. I thank you and praise you, Father. In Jesus' name...Amen.

*If the Holy Spirit is revealing sin in your life, please don't ignore Him. The way to health and healing begins with being honest with yourself and with God. It is the only way to truly change your life.

Day 21 - Your Body, God's Temple

1 Corinthians 3:16-17
Don't you know that you yourselves are God's temple and that God's spirit lives in you? If anyone destroys God's temple, God will destroy him; for God's temple is sacred, and you are that temple.

In the Old Testament, God's spirit dwelt in the Holy of Holies in His temple. God gave specific detailed instructions for the design and maintenance of Solomon's temple. If you read about it in the Bible, you will notice how impressively beautiful it was—like a glittering jewel displayed on a mount in the city of Jerusalem. By God's law, everything that entered that temple had to be pure and clean. God wanted pilgrims near and far to be irresistibly drawn to this holy place, and people only needed to look at it to realize that the temple was sacred ground where the God of the Universe met with his people.

After Jesus died for our sins, God placed His Holy Spirit in the believer in the same way that Jesus spoke of His own body being a temple (John 2:21). If you are a born-again child of God, then God's spirit resides in you. We no longer need to offer blood sacrifices in an earthly temple built of stone because Jesus was, and is, the ultimate sacrifice for our sins. We no longer need a high priest to enter the Holy of Holies on our behalf because Jesus is our High Priest, constantly interceding for us before the Lord. Because we are the temple of the Holy Spirit, we can personally commune with God anytime we want. What a privilege!

If we are the body-temple of God then how should we care for our human bodies, His holy dwelling place? First of all, we should address any habits or sins that are controlling our thoughts and actions and see them as God sees them. They are idols in His temple, and they need to go. Just as a basic starting point, we must pay careful attention to how we maintain our bodies. What food goes into your body? Is it real food? Is it pure or processed? Does your diet resemble the original diet God gave to mankind in Genesis 1:29? On this whole food plant-based diet, humans lived disease-free for the first 1,000 years on earth. It is interesting to note that the farther man has strayed from this original diet in Genesis 1 the sicker he has become.

Doctors today are finally telling us that what we eat does make a difference. Too much fat, sugar, and animal protein cause obesity, cancer, diabetes, heart disease, and strokes. Chemical additives and preservatives add a host of other ailments and allergies. Doesn't it stand to reason then, if we avoided these empty-calorie and fat-laden foods we would also avoid suffering the lifestyle diseases that go along with them—the plagues of modern times?

Are you eating 7 – 10 servings of vegetables and fruit every day? That is difficult to do only if you fill up on meat, dairy, and desserts. Are you drinking 6 – 8 glasses of pure water daily? Or, 6 – 8 cups of coffee with an occasional soda pop just to break the monotony? Only pure water flushes toxins from your body. Caffeinated and flavored acidic drinks add toxins that your body must work even harder to expel. If you want strong bones and teeth you must avoid soda.

God says that we reap what we sow (Galatians 6:7). That is a natural law we cannot deny. Even if we do not view the maintenance of our body temples as a sacred trust, God does, and He tells us that if we abuse His temple, we will be destroyed. That may sound harsh, but God hasn't changed the natural laws He set in place in the beginning simply because His people don't like them.

We cannot set up idols of food and drink in our lives and then expect God to bless us with robust health. That reasoning defies natural law, God's Word, and human logic. As Christians, we should not think we honor God by church attendance and Bible study (both good spiritual disciplines) if we neglect to properly nourish and care for the physical body in which His Holy Spirit resides.

How many churches are praying for revival and even teaching that revival starts with the individual? If we truly want to see revival in our churches, the gifts of the Holy Spirit moving in power as they did in days gone by, shouldn't we at least start by taking down the idols of food and drink in our personal lives? Instead, we joke about our caffeine and fast-food addictions so much that gluttony has become the only acceptable sin within the church. Let's clean up God's temple and strive to be healthy and pure in all areas, including our diets. This is not fanaticism; this is basic. It is a spiritual as well as a physical discipline, and surely disciples of the Lord must be disciplined.

In the Old Testament, we see the many times Israel suffered under bad kings who did evil in the sight of God, worshipped idols, and neglected God's temple. Eventually God's Spirit departed, and the people suffered years of misery. But when Israel repented, their loving Father forgave their sins and healed them. If we bring our eating habits under the discipline of God's Word as an act of submission to His lordship, eating the whole foods He originally designed for our well-being, our bodies will naturally heal themselves. That is God's blueprint for our health! He designed us so that healing is a natural process, but sickness is not. If we do our part by removing unhealthy idols from His temple, would health within the church, rather than sickness, become the norm? Would spiritual revival begin in the individual—in the church? Would Christians be a testimony to the world of God's healing grace and power? Would the world see and be drawn to the temple of the one true God?

BATTLE PLAN
CLEAN OUT YOUR PANTRY AND REFRIGERATOR

1. Be Ruthless! Do it now and you won't have temptation staring at you whenever you open the cupboard or refrigerator door. Fight for your health!

2. Be Honest! Ask yourself, "Is this really food (namely, nutrition for my body), or merely a manmade imitation of food?" Useless, empty calories (chips, pretzels, soda, candy, TV dinners, sugary breakfast cereals, white bread, and pastries) will only sabotage your efforts to strengthen your immune system and improve your health. Sugar and white flour, which your body processes as sugar, depress your immune system for hours!

3. Be Thrifty! Every dollar you spend on junk food is a dollar you won't have to purchase healthy real food. Research shows that when you consider cost per serving, whole plant foods are by far the better bargain. The reason people sometimes think eating healthy is expensive is that they are trying to support both a healthy and an unhealthy lifestyle at the same time, and that is expensive. In addition, buying healthy food does not cost more than doctor visits, prescriptions, surgery, and lost time at work. Don't rob yourself!

4. Be Wise! Be a label reader. Educate yourself on every food item you purchase. The fewer ingredients on the label the more natural and nutritious the product is. Hint: Whole fruits and vegetables have no ingredient labels—what you see is the only ingredient. When you see a paragraph of ingredients you don't recognize and can't even pronounce… BEWARE! Most of those extra ingredients are added to artificially improve appearance or

taste—in other words, to trick you into buying something you would never want to eat without the chemical disguise. It's just dressed up empty fat and calories.

5. Be Open-Minded! The only way to change your body is to change the habits that have gotten you to where you are today. You must be willing to part with that one favorite food you're clinging to, or you will never find a healthy substitute to replace it. If you insist on keeping a stock of dairy ice cream in the freezer you will never experiment with vegan ice cream recipes. If you continue to store soda and bottled juices then that is what you will reach for, and you will never switch to herbal tea, raw juices, and water.

6. Be Brave! Don't be afraid to change. You are stronger than you think. You can do this because your body is too important to ignore any longer. Your health will not change unless you change what you have been doing, so do it now. You are worth it!

Day 22 - The Proverbs 31 Wife

Proverbs 31:14-15, 26-27
She is like the merchant ships bringing her food from afar. She gets up while it is still dark; she provides food for her family and portions for her servant girls.... She speaks with wisdom, and faithful instruction is on her tongue. She watches over the affairs of her household and does not eat the bread of idleness.*

For years, every time I heard a sermon in church about "The Proverbs 31 Wife" I would fidget and squirm in my seat, counting the minutes until it would finally be over. The nerve of that preacher (usually a man) challenging us mere mortals to aspire to that superwoman ideal! I despised "The Proverbs 31 Wife," the perfect homemaker who makes even Martha Stewart look like a slacker. She made me feel like such a failure.

Then one day the Lord highlighted some of those verses in Proverbs 31 and spoke to my heart. "You are that woman —you are doing those things," He said.

"I am?" I read the verses again. I tried to understand what God was telling me.

Well, as I drove from health food store to grocery store to farmers' market, crisscrossing the county searching for the freshest produce and organic ingredients for my vegetarian recipes, I definitely was "bringing my food from afar." And while I normally don't "get up while it is still dark" (unless it's the middle of the winter when sunrise happens around 7:30 a.m. where we live), I do spend hours chopping, slicing, and dicing the freshest vegetables and fruits, testing, altering, and planning the healthiest and most nutritious plant-based meals I can prepare for my family.

A long time ago I realized that it does take extra time and effort to plan and prepare a healthy meal, but if we were going to walk this path to better health, I decided I would just do it anyway. Fresh salads must be made daily. Healthy natural foods, the way God designed them, do not come in a can or a plastic wrapper ready to pop into the microwave. However, if you invest the time it takes to eat properly, your body will reward you with better health and more energy almost immediately. Are you and your family worth the extra effort? Definitely – YOU ARE WORTH IT!

As far as speaking "with wisdom and faithful instruction," . . . well, you couldn't stop me. Learning what the Bible has to say about health and healing and the visible results I've seen in my own body have excited me almost as much as my salvation experience. It is hard not to share what I've learned with anyone who will sit still and listen. But I have noticed that more is caught than is taught, so I try not to overwhelm the people I love with my verbal zeal. Eating and serving healthy food is the best way to lead by example.

You have more influence over your family's eating habits than you realize, but they will be more willing to follow your daily example than to listen to you preaching at them. Children may not always do what you say, but like little sponges, they are always watching and learning from what you do. So, you lead the way in proper nutrition and healthy food choices in your family. For example, don't put your husband on a low cholesterol diet unless you are willing to eat the same things. That only leads to nagging, and it just will not work. Besides, if it's good for him, then it's good for you, too. You are the manager of your household. You determine what kinds of foods are in your pantry and refrigerator—healthy or unhealthy. If there are no hot dogs or hamburgers in the freezer, then you won't be tempted to serve them for supper. Your family will not snack on cookies, chips, and soda pop if they aren't in the house. Fruit is a wonderful snack: nutritious, sweet, and colorful. It even comes in its own edible or biodegradable wrapper and creates no dirty dishes to wash (gotta love that!). When your children see you munching a crunchy red apple or snacking on a handful of colorful berries or a thick slice of cold juicy watermelon, I promise they will want some, too!

So, do what it takes to guide your family into a healthy diet and lifestyle. Lead by example, and when you must, speak the truth in love. Soon your family will learn to appreciate, and even prefer, colorful, nutritious living foods and will choose these over dead, pre-packaged convenience foods. You can influence the health of future generations by setting a healthy example today.

Signed,

The Proverbs 31 Wife ;-)

*For the entire Bible passage about the Proverbs 31 Wife, please read Proverbs 31:10-31

BATTLE PLAN
EGG SUBSTITUTIONS

What do you do about eggs? Well, eggs are an animal food (think of them as liquid chicken) containing fat and cholesterol you really don't need. The shells are fragile and porous, and conditions on chicken farms are crowded and cruel. This makes eggs an ideal host for salmonella, a bacteria that is the leading cause of food poisoning. For these reasons, I don't keep eggs in the house and try to avoid eating them at all times. Yet I still cook and bake many recipes by using egg substitutes. Here are some of my favorite egg substitutes:

Baking:

- 1 Tbs. ground flaxseed + 3 Tbs. warm water (allow to sit a few minutes until mixture thickens) = 1 egg
- 1 oz. mashed tofu = 1 egg
- Ener-G Egg Replacer, a vegan powdered product found in health food stores (follow package directions).
- ½ banana or ¼ cup applesauce (for sweet baking only) = 1 egg

As a binder in veggie burgers or "meat" loaves:

- Rolled oats
- Bread crumbs
- Mashed potato
- A little whole grain flour

Day 23 - Count Your Blessings
Psalm 4:8
I will lie down and sleep and sleep in peace, O Lord, make me dwell in safety.

Did you know that the amount of time you spend sleeping and the quality of your sleep is directly related to your health? We, as a nation, have become a 24/7 society. Besides the normal stressors of work, family, the economy, politics, etc. we have now added Internet, e-mail, cell phones, and smart TV. Americans are plugged in and "on" all the time!

One study of almost 10,000 adults aged 32 – 49 showed that people who sleep less than 7 hours per night are significantly more likely to be obese. This is due to the fact that lack of sleep disrupts the hormones, gherlin and leptin, that regulate appetite. Could your late-night hours be causing you to retain those stubborn pounds you have been trying so hard to lose?

In addition to poor diet and lack of exercise, the Harvard-run Nurses Health Study links insufficient sleep to an increased risk of a list of major diseases including colon cancer, breast cancer, heart disease, and diabetes. This is because sleep disruption also disturbs the production of hormones that play a role in these diseases. Poor sleep also increases the level of inflammation within the body creating an ideal environment for disease to develop and thrive.

Deprive yourself of sleep and you deprive your cells the opportunity to recover from the stresses of the day, repair damage and replicate healthy new cells.

Do you wonder why you seem to catch every cold or "bug" that is going around? Experts agree that 7 – 9 hours of quality sleep, not worrying about the past day or planning tomorrow's to-do list, is ideal. If you are getting less than 6 hours of peaceful sleep at night your immune system is exhausted, and you are three times more likely to develop the common cold. Less than 6 hours of sleep over a prolonged period of time even increases your risk of premature death.

Studies reveal that people who work at night are more prone than the general population to breast and colon cancer. This is believed to be related to decreased melatonin production within the body. Melatonin is a cancer fighting hormone that can only be produced while you sleep. Exposure to light at night greatly decreases your body's ability to produce melatonin. If you have a choice, it is better not to work at night, and when you do go to sleep keep the TV off and the room dark. Even the glow of a television or computer screen will interfere with melatonin production.

So, how do you start a routine that guarantees a good night's sleep? First of all, turn off and unplug! Make this your mantra. Your sleep is too important to be disturbed by phone calls, e-mails, flashing alarms, and beeping reminders. Turn off all electronic devices at least one hour before you plan to go to bed. Give your brain some uninterrupted time to wind down from the busyness of the day. Turn off the TV and radio! You don't need to hear the news one more time today; you can read or hear all about it tomorrow. Shut down your computer! It may take some practice before this routine feels comfortable, especially if you are used to constant electronic contact and background noise, but try. Soon you will begin to look forward to that moment when the buzz stops and all is quiet and peaceful in your world.

Still having trouble turning off your brain? Can't stop thinking about tomorrow or rehearsing what went wrong today? Don't count sheep—try praising! When was the last time you talked to God with no agenda and no fear of interruption? I don't mean praying over your list of wants and needs which can circle right back to worrying. As you lie there in the still darkness simply thank Him for everything that comes to mind...praise Him for who He is and all His blessings in your life. Thank Him for a warm bed, strength for the day, the opportunity to have a peaceful night's slumber, a heart that continues to beat, and lungs that breathe without a thought on your part. Thank Him for a body that is repairing itself and getting stronger even while you sleep. I promise, counting your blessings will help you to fall asleep in an attitude of gratitude that will help you to sleep soundly and wake refreshed. We need to remember the old Sunday School song that goes:

"Count your blessings, name them one by one. Count your many blessings, see what God has done!"

BATTLE PLAN
FOR MORE INFORMATION ABOUT SLEEP

healthysleep.med.harvard.edu/need-sleep/whats-in-it-for-you/health

Day 24 - Lordship

Romans 14:2-4, 17-18

One man's faith allows him to eat everything, but another man, whose faith is weak, eats only vegetables. The man who eats everything must not look down on him who does not, and the man who does not must not condemn the man who does, for God has accepted him. Who are you to judge someone else's servant? To his own master he stands or falls. And he will stand, for the Lord is able to make him stand.... For the kingdom of God is not a matter of eating and drinking, but of righteousness, peace and joy in the Holy Spirit, because anyone who serves Christ in this way is pleasing to God and approved by men.

The Bible is clear on this fact: our salvation does not depend on our eating habits. Our salvation depends on belief in Jesus Christ as the ultimate sacrificial Lamb of God, whose blood was shed on the cross to cover our sins. If we have faith in Jesus, we are saved—nothing more, nothing less.

I have heard Christians argue this point endlessly, each one trying to prove the other wrong, and Romans 14:2 is often quoted. Is it Biblical to be a vegetarian? Is it merely a New Age practice? Does God approve or condemn dietary restrictions? Scripture teaches us that we are not to condemn anyone for what he eats. Surely, we are not the Holy Spirit, and we have no right to judge our brothers and sisters even if we disagree on this topic. Besides, no one is ever won over by being criticized or put down in an argument just to prove that they are wrong and you are right; so please, resist that temptation. If you are concerned about the path another Christian is on, then pray that the Holy Spirit will convict them about their own health issues and nudge them in the right direction. Remember, unless someone asks for your advice they don't want it and aren't ready to listen. Until then, pray and be a witness of God's love and grace to them.

However, at some point in every Christian's life, the Holy Spirit confronts each one of us with the issue of "Lordship." When I was about twenty years old, the Lord started to convict me about wearing blue jeans. I was part of the hippie generation. At that time, all my friends and I thought it was cool to wear tattered blue jeans every day and for every occasion. (I would actually buy new jeans, gently slice all the seams and hems with a razor blade and then launder them several times so they were well faded and frayed before I ever wore them out in public). Well, one day the Lord spoke to my spirit and said, "My children don't dress this way. This is the uniform of failure." Ouch! God doesn't waste words, and He can be very efficient when dealing with our vices. Because I loved the Lord, I did give up wearing blue jeans for two whole years. As I was sensitive to His leading, He showed me how to dress, and to enjoy dressing like a successful adult. When I had finally learned that lesson, I felt released from the restriction. Today I do wear blue jeans; at the proper place and time, and they are not faded and frayed (I call those rags!)

God teaches each individual different lessons at different times in their personal Christian walk. It is at this point of discipleship that we see one man give up his lifelong career and head to Bible College to study for the ministry. A couple feels called to uproot their entire family and become missionaries in a foreign land. Another couple decides that it might be a financial and emotional stretch, but they obediently follow the Lord's leading and become foster parents to troubled kids. R. G. LeTourneau was called by God to give ninety percent of his income to Christian causes and to live on only ten percent. God wants to be alone on our heart's throne—to be our Lord and not merely our Savior. Only He knows the idols we are clinging to, and when He starts to clean house we often witness surprising and dramatic changes in our life and even our diet.

For many Americans food is an idol. We gorge at every meal and snack our way through the day with a cup of coffee always within arm's reach. Some adults are as cranky as a baby without her bottle if they can't get regular jolts of caffeine throughout the day! God may be dealing with you about your eating habits or your food addictions. Are you convicted about your diet? Do you control it, or does it control you? Is food one of your idols?

When we have false idols on our heart's throne, we are always disappointed because they never deliver the benefits we desire. Someone who makes financial success an idol may find herself entrenched and overextended in an unsatisfying career just for the money she can make there. A person who lives each day only to please herself may find she has only superficial personal relationships but no true friends she can really count on. With this emotional stress, we reap a harvest of physical illnesses: high blood pressure, ulcers, arthritis, autoimmune diseases, and cancer to name just a few. If you also struggle with food issues, you can add to that list high cholesterol, obesity, adult-onset diabetes, heart disease, and more.

False idols offer false hope. Only putting God first and making Him the Lord of your life will give you peace of mind and sound sleep at night. He may ask you to make some changes—to do some things differently. No need to worry; God is in control, and you can trust him. If He leads you to leave one job, He's able to provide a better job. If He asks you to give money to a worthy cause, He's able to provide more. If He guides you to give up an unhealthy diet and eat the designer foods He created, you will see weight come off and health problems disappear. Don't think of it as "giving up" anything! Your decision to eat only healthy foods will be the start of an exciting adventure as you discover colorful and delicious new foods you never even knew existed before you decided to transform your diet. You will be in better condition than you were if you submit to Him and smash your food idols. You will come to love healthy eating, and you will also love the way you look and feel as a result of your obedience to your Lord.

Our salvation does not depend upon whether or not we eat meat. Our eternal life is secured by our faith in Christ and nothing else. However, the quality of our life here and now on planet Earth is greatly dependent upon who or what is in control of our diet. Don't judge others, but examine your own walk with the Lord and ask yourself, "Are there any idols in my life? Is my diet out of control? Is food my idol?" Be honest. What do you think God wants you to do about that?

BATTLE PLAN
NINJA TUNA SALAD

This recipe makes a great summer, picnic, or take-to-work lunch. The flavor is better if made ahead, so make it the night before and preparing lunch the next day will be simple. (The secret ingredient is the nori – for real seafood flavor it makes all the difference in the world!)

1 16 oz. can (or 2 cups cooked) chickpeas, rinsed and drained

2 scallions, chopped

2 stalks celery, chopped

1 parsnip or carrot, finely shredded

½ - ¾ cup Vegenaise (or any other vegan mayo)

1 sheet nori (sushi wrapper sea vegetable), use scissors to snip into tiny thin pieces

1 tsp kelp granules

Sea salt and freshly ground pepper, to taste

A tsp. lemon juice, optional

*Organic ingredients are always preferred

Directions:

Place chickpeas in food processor and pulse until coarsely chopped (not pureed). If you don't have a food processor, you can use a good old-fashioned potato masher to mash them up.

Transfer to a large bowl.

Add all other prepared ingredients to the chickpeas and use a large spoon to mix everything together.

Refrigerate until served.

Serve a scoop of Ninja Tuna Salad on a bed of salad greens with tomato wedges or as a sandwich spread on whole grain bread. Makes 6 or more generous sandwiches.

Day 25 - Your Daily Bread

Ezekiel 4:9

"Take wheat and barley, beans and lentils, millet and spelt; put them in a storage jar and use them to make bread for yourself."

When my grandmother came to America, at the age of twenty, she fell in love with white bread. She called it "cake" because in the early 1900s in her Ukrainian homeland, there was no white flour for peasants; white flour was strictly for the wealthy. The only bread she had ever eaten until arriving in the United States was made with dark whole grain flour. In America, however, she made her fluffy white bread every week, along with lots of white noodly dishes.

Oh, she truly had come to The Promised Land!

In the last century, all of American society bought into the myth that white flour was better, more attractive, and to be preferred over dark. Certainly we were more affluent than ever before, so we should be able to eat like the rich—we'd earned it; we deserved "the best!"

Little did my grandmother realize that the dark bread she grew eating in the "Old Country" was really the best for her body. Whole grains are an important part of a healthy diet. The keyword here is "whole." When buying bread, you should always look for a label that says "whole grain bread," not one that merely "contains whole grain," because the portion of whole grains it contains may actually be very small indeed. If the bread has a light and fluffy texture, similar to foam rubber, it's not the bread you want. Look for a heavy dense loaf with a bit of a chewy "crunch" to the crust.

Refined grains are almost fiberless, causing constipation, which is a chronic problem in America. Think of the flour and water paste (papier mache) you used to make in elementary school and realize that your digestive system is clogged with this gloppy gunk every time you eat white bread, pasta, or any bakery item made from refined white flour. When purchasing bread, don't just look at the color. Some companies use molasses to tint their baked goods so they look like they are made with dark whole grains. Reading the ingredients listed on the package, not just the front label, is the only way to be sure that the first ingredients are whole grain flours.

Refined grains are quickly broken down into sugar in the body, causing diabetic/hypoglycemic reactions and suppression of the immune system. These refined, empty calories are also acid-forming. Acidity within the body creates inflammation. To neutralize the acid, your body efficiently extracts calcium from your bones, contributing to osteoporosis! Who wants that?

Look at the grains mentioned in Ezekiel 4:9. God has given us many more grains than just wheat to meet our nutritional needs. Why have we Americans limited our diets to rely so heavily on that single grain? Let me challenge you to try some of the others. Millet, spelt, barley, oats, quinoa, amaranth, and others can be found in health food stores and even in some grocery stores. Try some of these different whole grains cooked or soaked overnight for breakfast. How about swapping your white rice for brown rice tonight for dinner? You will be amazed by how satisfying and filling it is. Because brown rice has the bran intact, it is more nutritious and less constipating than white rice. You can even find flours made from legumes (notice that beans and lentils were included in Ezekiel's bread) and baked goods made from sprouted grains in some stores today. When buying grains, remember organic grains and flours are always the best. Any grain that is genetically modified or chemically contaminated is not recommended for a healthy diet.

Be adventurous. Don't be afraid to try new grains. Some of these grains are quite ancient and even predate wheat in the human diet. You are not familiar with them because they are not common in the Standard American Diet. You can find many good recipes online. Simply do an Internet search for recipes including whatever grain you desire, and then experiment with a few of the many dozens of recipes you find. These grains are just as versatile as wheat—you've just never tried them before.

Keep in mind that when God told Ezekiel the ingredients to put in his bread, that bread had to contain enough life-sustaining nutrients to support him for the 390 + 40 days (more than a year!) Ezekiel had to lie on his side to illustrate God's prophecy to His people (Ezekiel 4:9-17). God was calling Ezekiel to do something big for Him, and his diet was a critical part of the task. God didn't tell him to eat bleached white flour, white rice, or sugar during that time. The ingredients in Ezekiel's bread supplied enough nutrition to complete the assignment God gave him to do. What is God asking you to do? Are you eating to complete the task?

BATTLE PLAN
OVERNIGHT CHAI STEEL-CUT OATS

This is a chai-flavored breakfast recipe that I absolutely love. It's so great because you put it all together the night before, and in the morning it's ready to eat ... no cooking time!

1 c. steel-cut oats

1 c. non-dairy "milk"

2 Tbs. chia seeds

1/4 tsp. ground cardamom

1/4 tsp. vanilla

1/4 tsp. ground ginger or 1 Tbs. chopped crystallized ginger (Crystal-lized ginger tastes amazing... spicy sweet with a tangy bite).

1/4 tsp. ground cinnamon

1 pinch nutmeg

1 pinch black pepper

1 Tbs. maple syrup

1 Tbs. shredded coconut, optional

1 Tbs. chopped pistachios, optional

Directions:

Combine first ten ingredients in a glass jar with a lid (a canning jar works fine). Stir, close lid, and refrigerate overnight.

Next day:

Add as much non-dairy milk as desired, stir, then put each serving into a bowl and top with coconut and pistachios, if using. (You may warm it slightly before eating if you like).

Day 26 - The Best Medicine

Proverbs 17:22
A merry heart does good like a medicine, but a broken spirit dries up the bones.

Have you ever met someone whose smile just lights up the room? Someone whose mere presence attracts and encourages others? We all know people who despite physical illness, depressing family circumstances, or personal loss still manage to greet each day with a positive attitude and a kind word for others. The very atmosphere around these people seems positively charged as they spread warmth and light wherever they go. We also know others who complain about every little thing in life and manage to turn each conversation into a gripe session about the economy, politics, their boss, husband, children, etc.; something always irritates them, and in their eyes society, in general, is teetering on the brink of disaster. These people leave doom, gloom, and despair in their wake. We usually try to avoid being cornered by such people because it's impossible to escape their negative state of mind—even changing the subject doesn't help for very long because they will soon think of something else to grumble about.

What is the difference between these two types of personalities? The positive person has learned that real joy doesn't come from our circumstances but from within and ultimately from the Lord who lives in us, rather than from what is happening around us. Nothing can steal real joy. If you are focused only on yourself and your own circumstances, then having a merry heart may take great effort. For emotional health, you must strive to break away from the handcuffs of negative thought and speech. Remind yourself of the Father's great love for you and all the blessings you do have. (Come on—you're alive and living in a free country, plus you have eternity in Heaven to look forward to—you ARE blessed!) When we acknowledge the blessings we do have, instead of focusing on what we lack, we give ourselves permission to smile and even laugh.

It feels so good to be free in your spirit instead of wrapped in the chains of negativity. Research has proven that laughter lowers blood pressure, relieves stress, releases endorphins (the body's natural pain killers), and activates the immune system. All these things help your body to heal itself naturally. I have even heard doctors claim that they can almost predict if a patient will recover by that patient's attitude. This proves a strong spirit/body connection we cannot deny. Negativity is one bad habit you must conquer. You will not have a healthy physical body if you choose to live with a negative attitude. It really is healing to laugh, even at yourself!

So, how can you foster a positive, joyful spirit? One way is through prayer. Pray and thank God for everything you can think of. You can even thank Him for the not-so-good things that happen. I have a friend who does this all the time. Whenever a problem arises he says with a smile, "Praise God, another chance for Him to increase and me to decrease," or "Thank you, Lord, for another opportunity for me to be weak and You to be strong." When I first heard my friend talk this way, I was shocked that he could be so calm in the face of what would clearly be seen by most people as a major setback. I soon learned, however, that he was speaking from a deep inner conviction that in the Lord's hands, his future would be all right, and he was trusting God to take care of the details along the way. With this conscious attitude adjustment, my friend can relax and smile even in difficult situations.

A merry heart does not happen by mere chance or good fortune. We must actively choose, as my friend does, to focus on what is positive and uplifting and purposefully filter out the fearful negative pressures around us. Decide to forgo the nightly news and instead watch something on television that makes you laugh—you will feel so much better! Read inspirational books and listen to quality music. Choose to surround yourself with happy, motivated people and loving relationships. When you are tempted to contribute to a negative conversation, stop and think of something positive and encouraging to say instead. Resolve to simply avoid people who are complaining and critical. Don't worry about offending those Negative Nellies. When you refuse to participate in their pessimism, then they will soon begin to avoid you!

Decide to "be of good cheer." Jesus has overcome the world, and even if circumstances do not change, you can live victoriously in any situation with His help. Foster an attitude of gratitude; there is always, always something to be grateful for. Thank God and choose to enjoy this gift called life! For heaven's sake, step outside yourself and discover how you can help someone else. Which neighbor needs a little help? Which organization is looking for volunteers? Do you know someone who is sick and could use a visit or a phone call? What can you do? At the very least you can always pray for someone else's needs. It is hard to feel sorry for yourself when you are focused on the welfare of others.

Please, embrace every opportunity to smile and laugh; go out and find them! Before long you will become that positive person that lights up the room. You will soon come to realize that a merry heart is better than any medicine money can buy!

BATTLE PLAN
LAUGH YOUR WAY TO HEALTH

Everyone enjoys a good laugh. Remember when you were a child, laughing so hard that your stomach hurt and you could hardly catch your breath? That kind of deep belly laugh is actually healing, so make laughter a new habit! Here are some hilarious Christian comedians you can find on CD, DVD, or on www.youtube.com:

- Bob Smiley
- Chonda Pierce
- Dennis Swanberg
- Mark Lowry
- Tim Hawkins

Laughter is the best medicine, so chuckle, giggle, fall on the floor, and roar with laughter—just have a good time!

Day 27 - Conform or Transform

Romans 12:1-2

Therefore, I urge you, brothers, in view of God's mercy, to offer your bodies as living sacrifices, holy and pleasing to God – this is your spiritual act of worship. Do not conform any longer to the pattern of this world, but be transformed by the renewing of your mind. Then you will be able to test and approve what God's will is – His good, pleasing and perfect will.

Wouldn't it be wonderful if everyone who prayed for healing was instantly zapped from above with perfect health, a fit and trim physique, shiny hair, and dazzling white teeth? We'd love that miraculous cure for whatever ails us in this fast-paced, get-it-done-now society in which we live. Imagine it: You go up to the altar, pray for healing, and zap—you're healed!... Next? It just doesn't happen that way, though. Instead, church altars are lined every week with the same believers seeking prayer for healing, and our personal prayer lists are mostly roll calls of the sick people we know?

Sadly, many of those praying for healing will never get well. A lot of people live in dread of their next lab report or doctor appointment, feeling that the odds are against them ever regaining their health or strength. They fear their survival depends on the coin toss of chance unless God miraculously intervenes.

Does God still heal today? Definitely! So why isn't everyone who prays for healing being healed? Why are so many disappointed when their prayers seem to go unanswered? Could it be that God is asking His people to do something more in the process? Are we taking our body to the altar for healing prayer like we take our car into the service center—only when it won't start or when it's making a funny clinking noise?

If we are to present our bodies as "living sacrifices," then it is our sacred duty to do everything we can to ensure the health of these bodies every day, not just when we get sick. We shouldn't mindlessly live as though how we care for our bodies doesn't matter—it does! Old Testament sacrifices were perfect, without spot or blemish. Are we? Are the bodies we present as living sacrifices to the Lord well maintained, or overfed but undernourished; overweight and under-exercised; young in years, but already worn out from overuse and hard living?

In the Bible, animals designated for sacrifice were exceptional. The farmer carefully inspected each animal in his flock or herd. Only the very best, the healthiest County Fair Blue Ribbon Champion, was chosen for sacrifice. That animal was guarded, protected, and daily fed a superior diet by its owner. Only a perfect specimen was deemed worthy to be sacrificed to the Holy God of Israel.

This is an object lesson for all of us. As we present our bodies to be living sacrifices, do we honor God by offering Him the very best we can be, or do we offer a sick, tired, overweight, worn-out body? Are we living like the world, and then placing this weak left-over sacrifice on the altar of the living God? Is this true worship?

Believers must take action. To our shame, diet seems to be the one area of life the church has decided does not fall under the lordship of Christ. To be a worthy sacrifice, we must treat our physical bodies as an offering to our Lord. We must choose to eat the whole natural foods God created for the superior health man enjoyed in The Garden instead of mindlessly gorging on processed substitutes which provide no real nutrition. It may not be easy to choose fresh green broccoli over greasy salty french fries, but do it anyway as an act of spiritual submission and of worship.

Every time you eat an apple instead of a doughnut, drink water rather than soda pop, or order a vegetable stir-fry instead of roast beef or fried chicken for dinner, you are declaring to yourself and the world, "He is Lord over every aspect of my life." This may not be the way you are used to eating. It may not be the way your friends and family eat. That is irrelevant. The fact is that Christians are supposed to be different. We can't eat like the world and expect to live in divine health. We are not called to "conform to this world"—that's what we did in our former lives. Now we are to "be transformed by the renewing of our minds."

As we learn what God says about diet and lifestyle, we will make better choices for maintaining health. We will be transformed. This is a physical and a spiritual process. As a butterfly emerges from the cocoon and unfolds its wings, the results of your submission to your Lord and King in the areas of diet, exercise, thought life, relationships, etc. will soon prove that God's perfect will is superior physical and emotional health and vitality. Your metamorphosis, just as the butterfly's, will be evident to you and everyone around you.

Am I saying that changing your diet and lifestyle habits will guarantee healing? Not necessarily. But, if you properly nourish and care for your physical body every day, then you will definitely improve your immune system's ability to fight back and recover from any illness. Why would you deliberately sabotage your body's natural healing process with an unhealthy diet? Animal foods, sugar, high-fat fast foods, chemically-laden junk foods—these place enormous stress on a sick body as it tries to process them at the very time the body desperately needs all its energy to fight illness and regain strength. So, every day, do everything within your power to maintain a healthy body. Don't wait until you get sick to try and turn things around. It will only be harder then. Start now. God has already given you a wonderful self-healing body—cooperate with Him on this!

BATTLE PLAN
TAKE THE INITIATIVE

The first step is yours, and no one can take it for you. Find a vegetarian, vegan, or raw food cooking class, and sign up NOW! If you don't know of any, then inquire at your health food store or local chiropractor's office. Your health is worth the investment. You probably spend more on one appointment at the hairdresser for only temporary outward improvement, but a good vegan cooking class will give you the tools you can use for a lifetime of health and healing on the inside. At a cooking class, you will meet new friends, and you will soon have a collection of delicious recipes you are confident in preparing.

When you develop a group of like-minded friends, host a vegan potluck. Make it a regular monthly event! Share your ideas and recipes. Watch a health-related video or do a book study together. You will all be more successful as you support and encourage each other on the road to better health.

Day 28 - Honey Dos and Dont's

Proverbs 24:13, 25:16,27
Eat honey, my son, for it is good; honey from the comb is sweet to your taste... If you find honey, eat just enough – too much of it and you will vomit... It is not good to eat too much honey...

When we think of any kind of diet, trimming calories, or losing weight, the first thing most people try to do is restrict their consumption of sugar. Even though sugar is only empty calories, and we really can live without it, sugar is also undeniably extremely addictive. Most children are introduced to sugar at an early age, and those cravings stay with them forever.

Sugar consumption in the United States has skyrocketed since records were first kept in 1822. At that time, the typical American consumed the amount of sugar found in one of today's 12 oz. cans of soda every five days. That amount has ballooned 17 times to a whopping 130 pounds of sugar per year consumed by the typical American. Modern adults are now eating 22 tsp. of sugar per day, and the average child in this country consumes even more – 32 tsp. per day! This translates into an extra 500 calories every day—the equivalent of 10 strips of fatty bacon! White table sugar is not the only problem. High fructose corn syrup is in almost every processed food on the market from breakfast cereals to ketchup. Is it any wonder that we, as a nation, are the heaviest we've ever been?

Unlike fruit, which contains natural sugar, these highly processed, concentrated sugars contain no fiber to slow down the absorption. Your liver will step up bile production to process all this concentrated sugar just like it would for alcohol. With this day after day sugar saturation, it's easy to overload your liver and drive the progress of insulin resistance. This sets the stage for chronic illnesses: obesity, heart disease, diabetes, and even liver disease.

Because excess sugar in the diet leads to weight gain, high blood pressure, and creates an acidic internal environment that actually feeds cancer, the American Heart Association recommends no more than 6 tsp. per day for women and 9 tsp. for men. This means cutting your sugar consumption by about two-thirds. Are you up for the challenge?

Seeking an easy solution without sacrificing their sweet tooth, many people turn to artificial sweeteners. These harmless-looking pastel packets can be found everywhere from restaurant tables and coffee shops to hospital room lunch trays. Seems like a simple low-calorie solution, right? Wrong!

The words "artificial," "substitute," or "diet" on any package should be a clue. Our bodies are designed to recognize only real foods as God created them. Chemically altered food substitutes are regarded as toxins by your liver, which ramps up bile production to flush these toxins out of your body. This in turn interferes with your liver's ability to process fats, its main function, and leads to guess what—weight gain! It's true; sugar substitutes make you fat! And because artificial sweeteners are much sweeter than sugar, they reinforce your sweet tooth with even stronger sugar cravings. Every single artificial sweetener has been linked to adverse biological reactions, so if you are wise, you won't subject your body to those hazardous chemicals. You may ask why these products are being sold if they aren't safe. Remember, the companies that create and market these products are also the companies that test them, and test procedures can be manipulated and results interpreted to mean almost anything, especially if there is a financial incentive.

By now you are probably wondering what sweetener is safe to use. Raw, unfiltered honey is the natural sweetener provided by God and recommended in His Word. Raw honey contains the many benefits of vitamins, minerals, and enzymes not present in refined, sometimes labeled "Fancy" honey, the kind normally found in grocery stores. The best place to get raw, unfiltered honey is directly from a beekeeper or at your local farmers' market or health food store.

The healing powers of honey are legend. Raw, unfiltered honey has antibacterial and antifungal properties. In general, the darker the honey the greater its antibacterial and antifungal power. Local honey can even eliminate seasonal allergies as you become desensitized to the minute amounts of pollen the honey from your geographic area contains. Manuka honey is sometimes used to treat leg ulcers and pressure sores, and new research claims it may even be an effective weapon against MRSA infections.

Remember, sugar is sugar, and too much of any type of sugar is not good. This includes carbohydrates such as potatoes and grains which are processed like sugar in the body. If you are diabetic, this is non-negotiable. Sugar is not a necessary ingredient in our diet; it's just a habit. We must take control of our sugar cravings instead of feeding them. Make sugar an occasional treat instead of an idol—an every day, all the time addiction. Your body will thank you.

BATTLE PLAN
HONEY AS MEDICINE

Sore throat: A little honey and lemon in warm water is a soothing drink to calm a scratchy throat.

Coughs: In a study of 110 children, a single dose of buckwheat honey was just as effective as a single dose of dextromethorphan (cough syrup) in relieving nighttime coughs and allowing them to sleep.*

Seasonal allergies: Starting a few months prior to allergy season, take one tsp. local raw honey several times per day to gradually desensitize yourself to pollens in your area. Continue this process daily.

*Caution: NEVER give honey to children under one year old because their immature immune systems can't defend against botulism bacteria in the dust and soil that may make its way into the honey.

Day 29 - Shopping In the Garden

Proverbs 6:6-8, 30:25
Go to the ant, you sluggard; consider its ways and be wise! It has no commander, no overseer or ruler, yet it stores its provisions in summer and gathers its food at harvest. ...Ants are creatures of little strength yet they store up their food in the summer.

If you have even a little bit of land, I encourage you to plant a garden. It doesn't take much space to hold a few tomato plants, some zucchini, and radishes. Growing your own will ensure that your garden produce is totally organic—what a money saver! Plus, it is relaxing for the mind and exercise for the body to be out in the sunshine digging in the soil and savoring the beauty of nature. As you watch the tiny seeds you plant sprout, grow, and finally blossom into a bountiful harvest, you will be blessed with a front-row seat to observe God's plan and provision for feeding His supreme creation: humankind.

In our home gardening, canning, and freezing our own garden produce has always been a family affair. Even the youngest child can learn to identify and pull weeds, dig a hole to bury compost, shell peas, and husk corn. If everyone works together, it becomes a hobby, not a chore. I have even witnessed a picky young eater who wouldn't touch a cooked vegetable under threat of death at the supper table, wander through the garden grazing on fresh snap peas and green beans. Kids seem to instinctively prefer crunchy, raw veggies and think of them as snacks. Knowing that they helped grow the vegetables makes them even more appealing in a child's eyes.

If your garden is small, or for more variety, you can shop at your local farmers' market. Even non-organic, local produce is fresher and has not been sprayed as much as produce that is trucked cross-country or imported. Most city dwellers have access to at least one farmers' market. You can find great deals at the end of the day at many markets if you are willing to buy large quantities at greatly discounted prices. Fruits and vegetables are perishable, so farmers would rather sell their leftover produce at a reduced cost than pack it up, transport it back to the farm, and have it spoil anyway. If you don't see advertised mark-downs at the end of the day, ask. Don't worry about buying more than you can use. Maybe you can share with a friend. You can get instructions online for freezing, canning, or dehydrating your bargains, or you can call your County Extension Office and they will send the information to you. This is a wonderful way to stretch your food dollars and improve your family's diet! When the winter storms come, it is so satisfying to see your pantry and freezer full of the beautiful fruits and vegetables you thought ahead to preserve.

A fun family outing is picking strawberries, blueberries, or cherries at a local farm. You pick as much as you want and pay by the pound—normally at a price that is much lower than what the grocery stores charge. Children love to eat what they pick. Looking at their round tummies and stained fingers and faces, it's a good thing farms don't weigh each child before and after picking and charge for those pounds, too! Making this a fun family event is a simple way to encourage kids to eat fresh whole foods as snacks.

In the fall, we have an annual family tradition of picking apples. Sometime in October we go to a local orchard and pick about 100 pounds of apples. (It really doesn't take long with everyone helping). There are many varieties of apples from which to choose, and you can sample them in the orchard to select the variety you like best.

We usually get one basket of Red and Golden Delicious for snacking, and a more tart variety for applesauce and pie filling. I love Jonathan and Black Twig (also called Arkansas Black) apples for making applesauce because they give the sauce a lovely pink color. Most apples store well if you keep them cold. Macintosh is a very tasty sweet/tart variety, but it's not a good keeper so don't pick those if you can't make your sauce or pie filling within the next week. (Having applesauce and pie filling made and frozen in advance will certainly lessen your stress during the winter holiday season!)

Let's not forget that God placed Adam and Eve in a garden because He wanted them to eat the fresh fruits and vegetables that grew there. It is no coincidence that fruits and vegetables are brightly colored, attractive to the eye, and easy to identify as something to be desired and consumed. God knew these were the perfect foods to nourish human beings, so He made them readily available. He wanted to attract Adam's and Eve's attention to the best nutrition to keep them healthy, so He made these plant foods inviting to all their senses.

I have heard people make the excuse that it costs too much to buy healthy food. Not if you do it God's way; smash that idol! It is fascinating that God mentions the lowly ant, one of His tiniest creatures, twice to illustrate the virtues of wisdom and thriftiness. So, enjoy the summer's bounty on your table, and like the ant, preserve and store your abundance for the long winter months ahead. All in all, gardening is fun, economical, relaxing, healthy, and productive— an educational experience on so many levels. It is highly recommended by your Creator!

BATTLE PLAN
HOW TO FREEZE RAW TOMATOES

Mmm, fresh garden tomatoes taste so much better than the puny bland varieties that grocery stores carry during the winter. Did you know that there is an easy way to preserve your extra summer tomatoes so you can enjoy them in recipes all winter? It doesn't take long, and it doesn't require any special skills or equipment. This is how it's done:

1. Wash and dry fresh ripe tomatoes and cut out the core (stem end).
2. Place cored tomatoes, blossom end down, on a baking sheet (do not allow them to touch each other), then place the entire tray in the freezer.
3. Freeze until solid, and then put frozen tomatoes into a gallon-size freezer bag. One bag can hold 5 or 6 average size tomatoes. Store them in the freezer until you want to use them in a recipe.
4. When ready to use just hold each tomato under hot running water for a few seconds until the skin cracks and easily slides off.
5. Set skinned tomatoes on a plate until they are slightly thawed and soften a bit (30 – 60 min)
6. Chop and use in your favorite recipe!

Day 30 - Blossom! Bloom! Grow!

Galatians 5:16, 22-24

So I say, live by the Spirit, and you will not gratify the desires of the sinful nature.... But the fruit of the Spirit is love, joy, peace, patience, kindness, goodness, faithfulness, gentleness, and self-control. Against such things there is no law. Those who belong to Christ Jesus have crucified the the sinful nature with its passions

Sometimes we like to think that the fruit of the Holy Spirit is automatic, like the gifts of the Holy Spirit. While it would be nice if God just zapped us one day and we had all the love, joy, peace, patience, kindness, goodness, faithfulness, gentleness, and self-control we would ever need, that's not quite the way it works. The Bible tells us that the gifts of the Spirit are individually given to believers, and He decides when and to whom (see 1 Corinthians 12:8-11). The fruit of the Spirit is another matter. Fruit must be nurtured, cultivated, and allowed to grow.

Think of it this way: if you brought a little peach tree home from the nursery, would you merely plop it into a hole in the backyard and never water it, never fertilize it, never stake it so that the trunk grew straight and sturdy? Would you never check it for pests or disease? After neglecting your little tree week after week, month after month, and year after year, do you really think you would be able to harvest luscious sweet peaches from it? Oh, you might get a few small wormy peaches from your neglected tree, but if you really want a bumper crop, then you must care for the fruit even before you see it. You must make it a priority to water, fertilize, and be alert for insect attacks and weather extremes. Good fruit doesn't just happen—you must work for it!

Like any other fruit, the fruit of the Spirit must be cultivated in order to grow well. How do you cultivate the fruit of the Spirit? By not gratifying the desires of the sinful nature! Notice that self-control is on that list of fruit Christians are to cultivate. Don't think that because it is last on the list that it is any less important than the others. In fact, self-control is at the heart of every other fruit of the Spirit. Do you really think you can have love, joy, peace, and all the rest if you don't practice self-control?

If you are a Christian, then the Holy Spirit lives in you and gives you the strength to resist temptation and practice self-control. You are not on a solitary walk through this life. You do not fight any battle alone, so don't believe that lie of the enemy ("I just don't have any self-control"—LIE!). God knew it would take some work; that's why He gave you a helper in the Holy Spirit. Sin should not control a Christian because you have the Holy Spirit advantage over other people in this world.

As you practice self-control in every area of life, you are watering and fertilizing your fruits of the Spirit. As you choose (yes, it is a choice) to be patient, loving, and kind, you are weeding out feelings of selfishness, bitterness, and anger. You cultivate patience and gentleness when you exercise self-control in dealing with your children, spouse, and co-workers. Do you see how it all works together? A self-controlled person is at peace with herself and with others.

In your physical body, you cultivate self-control and overcome the sin of gluttony by bringing your appetite into submission. If you desire to have a healthy, energetic body to minister for the Lord, or to achieve any goals you have set for yourself, then you must practice self-control in the areas of diet and lifestyle, too.

Pray, and the Holy Spirit will help you to make wise food choices, but you must be faithful. Be a discerning food shopper. If it isn't real food, don't even bring it into your house. There is a reason they call it "junk" food! The Holy Spirit cannot help you to eat right if there is only junk food in your pantry and hotdogs and ice cream in your freezer. You know what you need to do: cultivate the fruit of self-control! Practice self-control in your shopping, in your meal planning, when you eat out, and when you dine alone. You are in charge, so as a responsible adult, hold yourself accountable. As you cultivate self-control as a lifestyle, the fruit of the Spirit in every other area will begin to blossom, also. In addition, without all that junk food in your diet, you will begin to feel better almost immediately. This discipline is merely an exercise to prepare you for the even greater adventure the Lord has planned for your life. Don't settle for small wormy fruit—Blossom! Bloom! Grow!

BATTLE PLAN
SELF-CONTROL AT THE DINNER TABLE

1. Do not eat standing up. Set a place at the table with a placemat, dishes, napkin, and silverware. Make dinner time special even when dining alone.
2. Do not watch TV or read while you eat. Both activities will cause you to overeat because you aren't paying attention. Allow yourself to experience the meal.
3. Eat slowly. Savor and enjoy each mouthful as you chew it at least 12 times. This will help if you have any digestive issues because digestion begins with the enzymes in your mouth. It takes about 20 minutes for a feeling of satiety to set in. If you quickly gobble your food down in the first 5 minutes and proceed to second and third helpings, then in 20 minutes you may have already eaten way too much.
4. Put your fork down between bites and engage in polite dinner conversation. How was your day? What did you do? Do you need help with the dishes, your homework, etc.?
5. Most restaurant entrees are huge. When dining out ask your server to please box half your meal before serving it. You can enjoy the take-home portion the next day for lunch or dinner.
6. Dessert is unnecessary. Smash that idol! Make dessert, even healthy dessert, only an occasional treat (birthday party or company for dinner). Relax with a cup of tea or herbal coffee after your meal instead.

DAY 31 - His Benefits for Our Benefit

Psalm 103:2-5
Praise the Lord, O my soul, and forget not all His benefits — who forgives all your sins and heals all your diseases, who redeems your life from the pit and crowns you with love and compassion, who satisfies your desires with good things so that your youth is renewed like the eagle's.

Sometimes we look at life as a party and start to feel that as Christians we can't have any fun at the party because our Christian life consists of a list of "do nots" (thou shalt not this, that, or the other thing). We need to stop feeling sorry for ourselves and remember the benefits that are freely given to us as children of the King.

God forgives all our sins. For most of us, this alone is such a generous demonstration of His love and grace that we can barely comprehend it. If that weren't enough, He heals our diseases. All healing comes from God. Whether through medical treatments or faithful prayer, God has programmed our physical bodies to be self-healing with the proper care and nutrition. Isn't that amazing? A doctor may set your broken arm, but only God can knit the bones together again. A surgeon operates, but the incision heals because God has made our bodies to heal themselves. How miraculous! Scientists tell us that every day a healthy immune system fights off invading viruses, bacteria, and even cancers we are not aware of. We can observe this healing process every time we get a cut or scratch, and our body immediately forms a scab to cover the injury and protect the wound while healing takes place underneath. The only time this process doesn't work is when your immune system is in a weakened state, allowing toxic invaders to infiltrate and grow.

God created delicious, wholesome fresh fruits and vegetables in the beginning as the original and most nutritious diet for mankind. Yes, Adam and Eve were vegetarians. God didn't put the first humans in a butcher shop. He didn't put them in a bakery. It was not a coincidence that God placed the first man and woman in a garden where there was an abundant supply of the perfect foods they were physically designed to eat. On this natural plant-based diet, humans lived disease-free for the first one thousand years.

God wants to satisfy our desires with good things. How many times do we try to satisfy our desires with "not so good" or even "bad" things? When it comes to food, fresh is best. God did not create dead, chemically altered, sugar-coated, artificially colored "food"—man did. It has been said that if it comes in a cellophane wrapper or a cardboard box, then you shouldn't eat it. Fresh fruit comes in its own edible or biodegradable wrapper. You can't do better than that! Even a lot of "health foods" are merely man's attempt to improve on God's design. There is no "power" in most power bars. Those compressed, high-calorie bricks are packed with more fat and sugar than genuine nutrition and resemble candy bars more than anything else. The real power and pure nutrition are in whole, natural foods as God made them. The Creator knows best!

God not only forgives your sins. If you choose God's way of satisfying your appetite, your immune system will grow stronger. Eating refined sugar will cripple your immune system for the next four hours. It is not merely by chance that the winter flu season starts during the winter holidays when Americans are indulging in way too many sweet treats. If you want to avoid colds and flu wash your hands often and eliminate refined sugar and processed foods from your diet. If you are sick now, this is imperative. Sugar is very acidic, and a diet high in sugar consumption will create the perfect environment for disease to thrive.

He "redeems your life from the pit." Are you tired of living in the pits? Do you feel fatigued all the time? Are you depressed? No energy? Examine your diet. Smash that idol!

He "renews your youth." Do you want to feel younger? Do you want to have enough energy to play in the park with your children or grandchildren without huffing and puffing to catch your breath? Do you want to look younger, too? Eat most of your food raw, not cooked (dead). Living cells need living food to produce healthy new cells. Juicing fresh fruits and vegetables will help to increase your consumption of raw foods, and juices are an excellent source of immediate, concentrated nutrition.

Then, consciously choose the good things. Satisfy your desires with the natural nutrient-packed vegetables and fruits, legumes, seeds, nuts, and whole grains that God, in His creative love and wisdom, has provided. Don't cheat yourself by settling for the world's counterfeit instead of God's best. "And forget not all His benefits!"

BATTLE PLAN
APPLE PIE SMOOTHIE

When you crave a piece of good old-fashioned apple pie, you don't have to deny yourself. Try this quick and easy recipe. With much less fat and fewer calories than baked apple pie, it just might satisfy your craving!

1 cup almond milk*

1 peeled tart apple, cut up

½ tsp. cinnamon

1 tsp. ground flaxseed

Sprinkle of nutmeg

A couple of soaked pitted dates

Process: Place all ingredients in a blender, and blend until smooth and creamy.

*Hint: Use a cold apple straight from the refrigerator. Freeze your almond milk in ice cube trays and use those instead of unfrozen almond milk, then your smoothie will be even thicker and creamier.

"Dear children, keep yourselves from idols."
1 John 5:21

SAMPLE FOOD JOURNAL PAGE

BREAKFAST

LUNCH

DINNER

SNACKS

SAMPLE FOOD JOURNAL PAGE

BREAKFAST

LUNCH

DINNER

SNACKS

SAMPLE FOOD JOURNAL PAGE

BREAKFAST

LUNCH

DINNER

SNACKS

SAMPLE FOOD JOURNAL PAGE

BREAKFAST

LUNCH

DINNER

SNACKS

SAMPLE FOOD JOURNAL PAGE

BREAKFAST

LUNCH

DINNER

SNACKS

SAMPLE FOOD JOURNAL PAGE

BREAKFAST

LUNCH

DINNER

SNACKS

SAMPLE FOOD JOURNAL PAGE

BREAKFAST

LUNCH

DINNER

SNACKS

Made in United States
Troutdale, OR
09/17/2024

22921237R00095